Drug Hepatotoxicity

Editor

PIERRE M. GHOLAM

CLINICS IN
LIVER DISEASE

www.liver.theclinics.com

Consulting Editor
NORMAN GITLIN

February 2020 • Volume 24 • Number 1

ELSEVIER

1600 John F. Kennedy Boulevard • Suite 1800 • Philadelphia, Pennsylvania, 19103-2899

http://www.theclinics.com

CLINICS IN LIVER DISEASE Volume 24, Number 1
February 2020 ISSN 1089-3261, ISBN-13: 978-0-323-70857-9

Editor: Kerry Holland
Developmental Editor: Donald Mumford

Clinics in Liver Disease (ISSN 1089-3261) is published quarterly by Elsevier Inc., 360 Park Avenue South, New York, NY 10010-1710. Months of issue are February, May, August, and November. Business and Editorial Offices: 1600 John F. Kennedy Blvd., Ste. 1800, Philadelphia, PA 19103-2899. Customer Service Office: 3251 Riverport Lane, Maryland Heights, MO 63043. Periodicals postage paid at New York, NY and additional mailing offices. Subscription prices are $313.00 per year (U.S. individuals), $100.00 per year (U.S. student/resident), $572.00 per year (U.S. institutions), $409.00 per year (international individuals), $200.00 per year (international student/resident), $709.00 per year (international instituitions), $343.00 per year (Canadian individuals), $100.00 per year (Canadian student/resident), and $709.00 per year (Canadian institutions). Foreign air speed delivery is included in all *Clinics* subscription prices. All prices are subject to change without notice. **POSTMASTER:** Send address changes to *Clinics in Liver Disease*, Elsevier Health Sciences Division, Subscription Customer Service, 3251 Riverport Lane, Maryland Heights, MO 63043. **Customer Service: Telephone: 1-800-654-2452 (U.S. and Canada); 314-447-8871 (outside U.S. and Canada). Fax: 314-447-8029. E-mail: journalscustomer service-usa@elsevier.com (for print support); journalsonlinesupport-usa@elsevier.com (for online support).**

Reprints. For copies of 100 or more of articles in this publication, please contact the Commercial Reprints Department, Elsevier Inc., 360 Park Avenue South, New York, NY 10010-1710. Tel.: 212-633-3874; Fax: 212-633-3820; E-mail: reprints@elsevier.com.

Clinics in Liver Disease is covered in *MEDLINE/PubMed (Index Medicus)*, Science Citation Index Expanded, Journal Citation Reports/Science Edition, and Current Contents/Clinical Medicine.

Contributors

CONSULTING EDITOR

NORMAN GITLIN, MD, FRCP (LONDON), FRCPE (EDINBURGH), FAASLD, FACP, FACG
Head of Hepatology, Southern California Liver Centers, San Clemente, California, USA

EDITOR

PIERRE M. GHOLAM, MD, FAASLD
Professor of Medicine, Case Western Reserve University School of Medicine, Medical Director, Liver Center of Excellence, University Hospitals Cleveland Medical Center, Cleveland Ohio, USA

AUTHORS

RAÚL J. ANDRADE, MD, PhD
Unidad de Gestión Clínica de Aparato Digestivo, Instituto de Investigación Biomédica de Málaga-IBIMA, Hospital Universitario Virgen de la Victoria, Universidad de Málaga, Málaga, Spain, Centro de Investigación Biomédica en Red de Enfermedades Hepáticas y Digestivas (CIBERehd), Spain

MICHAEL BABICH, MD
Program Director, Department of Gastroenterology and Hepatology, Allegheny General Hospital, Allegheny Health Network, Pittsburgh, Pennsylvania, USA

EINAR S. BJÖRNSSON, MD, PhD
Professor, Department of Internal Medicine, Faculty of Medicine, Division of Gastroenterology and Hepatology, The National University Hospital of Iceland, University of Iceland, Reykjavík, Iceland

ALLYCE CAINES, MD
Transplant Hepatology Fellow, Henry Ford Hospital, Detroit, Michigan, USA

MANEERAT CHAYANUPATKUL, MD
Instructor, Department of Physiology, Division of Gastroenterology, Department of Medicine, Chulalongkorn University, Bangkok, Thailand

STANLEY MARTIN COHEN, MD, FAASLD, FACG
Medical Director of Hepatology, University Hospitals Cleveland Medical Center, Professor of Medicine, Case Western Reserve University School of Medicine, Digestive Health Institute, Cleveland, Ohio, USA

UMAR DARR, MD
Houston Methodist Medical Center, Houston, Texas, USA

BILLEL GASMI, MD
Clinical Associate, Laboratory of Pathology, National Cancer Institute, Bethesda, Maryland, USA

MEAGAN E. GRAY, MD
Division of Gastroenterology and Hepatology, The University of Alabama at Birmingham, Birmingham, Alabama, USA

NICHOLAS A. HOPPMANN, MD
Transplant Hepatology Fellow, Division of Gastroenterology and Hepatology, The University of Alabama at Birmingham, Birmingham, Alabama, USA

MARISA ISAACSON, MD
Gastroenterology Fellow, Department of Gastroenterology and Hepatology, Allegheny General Hospital, Allegheny Health Network, Pittsburgh, Pennsylvania, USA

DAVID E. KLEINER, MD, PhD
Senior Research Physician, Chief, Post-Mortem Section, Laboratory of Pathology, National Cancer Institute, Bethesda, Maryland, USA

BRENDAN M. McGUIRE, MD, MS
Division of Gastroenterology and Hepatology, The University of Alabama at Birmingham, Birmingham, Alabama, USA

LINDSAY MEURER, MD
Department of Internal Medicine, University Hospitals Cleveland Medical Center, Case Western Reserve University School of Medicine, Cleveland, Ohio, USA

DILIP MOONKA, MD, FAST, FAASLD
Medical Director of Liver Transplant, Henry Ford Hospital, Detroit, Michigan, USA

VICTOR NAVARRO, MD
Professor of Medicine, Einstein Medical Center, Philadelphia, Pennsylvania, USA

NAEMAT SANDHU, MD
Einstein Medical Center, Philadelphia, Pennsylvania, USA

THOMAS D. SCHIANO, MD
Division of Liver Diseases, Professor, Department of Medicine, Recanati/Miller Transplantation Institute, Icahn School of Medicine at Mount Sinai, New York, New York, USA

CAMILLA STEPHENS, PhD
Unidad de Gestión Clínica de Aparato Digestivo, Instituto de Investigación Biomédica de Málaga-IBIMA, Hospital Universitario Virgen de la Victoria, Universidad de Málaga, Málaga, Spain, Centro de Investigación Biomédica en Red de Enfermedades Hepáticas y Digestivas (CIBERehd), Spain

NORMAN LESLIE SUSSMAN, MD
Associate Professor of Medicine and Surgery, Baylor College of Medicine, Houston, Texas, USA

DEEPAK VENKAT, MD
Senior Staff Physician, Medical Director of Living Donor Transplant Program, Division of Gastroenterology and Hepatology, Department of Medicine, Henry Ford Hospital, Detroit, Michigan, USA

PAUL B. WATKINS, MD
Institute for Drug Safety Sciences, Eshelman School of Pharmacy, The University of North Carolina at Chapel Hill, Research Triangle Park, North Carolina, USA

JINYU ZHANG, MD
Gastroenterology Fellow, Division of Gastroenterology and Hepatology, Department of Medicine, Henry Ford Hospital, Detroit, Michigan, USA

ELIZABETH ZHENG, MD
Assistant Professor of Medicine, Columbia University Irving Medical Center, New York, New York, USA

Contents

Idiosyncratic drug-induced liver injury (DILI) is an underreported and underestimated adverse drug reaction. A recent population-based study found a crude incidence of approximately 19 cases per 100,000 a year. Amoxicillin-clavulanate continues to be the most commonly implicated agent in most Western countries, reported to occur in approximately 1 of 2300 users. In patients with drug-induced autoimmune hepatitis, liver tests often do not normalize with cessation of the drugs and require corticosteroids. DILI associated with jaundice can lead to death from liver failure or require liver transplantation in at least 10% of cases.

Identification of genetic predisposition to drug-induced liver injury (DILI) is of paramount importance. Early candidate gene studies have identified various polymorphisms in drug-metabolizing genes that infer increased DILI susceptibility. Few of these have been confirmed in more recent genome-wide association studies, which have identified several specific human leukocyte antigen (HLA) alleles. The low incidence rate of DILI, however, leads to a low positive predictive value for currently identified genetic variations, making them unsuitable for pre-prescription screening. HLA screening incorporated into clinical practice can aid the diagnostic process resulting in enhanced diagnostic accuracy and confidence.

Drug-induced liver injury is a diagnosis that relies on the patterns of injury associated with specific medications and toxins. The process by which a clinician determines which agent is the likely culprit of the liver injury is called causality assessment. The Roussel Uclaf Causality Assessment Method (RUCAM) and additional causality assessment methods have been developed with the goal of providing a more standardized, less subjective approach to causality assessment. RUCAM remains the most used standardized method, however many physicians continue to rely on their experience for causality assessment.

> Given the liver's role in drug metabolism, it is uniquely sensitive to potential drug-induced liver injury (DILI) despite inherent protective mechanisms. In this article, we focus on the most common causes of DILI and their patterns of injury. Although not comprehensive, we attempt to cover several classes of commonly used drugs, and their associated patterns of injury and management.

> The DILI-sim Initiative is a public-private partnership using quantitative systems toxicology to build a model (DILIsym) capable of understanding and predicting liver safety liabilities in drug candidates. The effort has provided insights into mechanisms underlying dose-dependent drug-induced liver injury (DILI) and interpatient differences in susceptibility to dose-dependent DILI. DILIsym may be useful in identifying drugs capable of causing idiosyncratic hepatotoxicity. DILIsym is used to optimize interpretation of traditional and newer serum biomarkers of DILI. DILIsym results are considered in drug development decisions. In the future, it may be possible to use DILsym predictions to justify reduction in size of some clinical trials.

> When patients with suspected drug-induced liver injury (DILI) undergo liver biopsy, the pathologist can provide a wealth of information on the morphologic changes. The most common histologic patterns of DILI include mimics of acute and chronic hepatitis as well as acute cholestasis, chronic cholestasis, and a mixed pattern that combines hepatitis with cholestasis. The pattern may suggest etiologies of injury or correlate with reported patterns of injury for specific agents. Biopsy may exonerate or indict particular drugs as causal agents of injury and provide specific information on severity of injury and specific types of changes related to various outcomes.

> Drug-induced liver injury (DILI) is the most common cause of acute liver failure (ALF) in Western countries. Without liver transplantation, the mortality rate for ALF approaches greater than 80%. Acetaminophen-related ALF may be associated with a rapid progression but fortunately has a high chance for spontaneous survival compared with idiosyncratic DILI–related ALF. Several prognostic scoring systems for severe DILI have been developed to aid clinicians in selecting patients who require urgent liver transplantation. Patients who undergo liver transplantation for ALF are at risk for early graft loss and death and should be closely followed.

Drug-induced liver injury (DILI) is an uncommon but significant cause of liver injury and need for liver transplant. DILI in the setting of chronic liver disease (CLD) is poorly understood. Clinical features of patients presenting with DILI in the setting of CLD are similar to those without CLD with the exception of a higher incidence of diabetes among those with CLD and DILI. Diagnosis of DILI in CLD is difficult because there are no objective biomarkers and current causality assessments have not been studied in this population. Differentiating DILI from exacerbation of underlying liver disease is even more challenging.

The hydroxymethyglutaryl-coenzyme A reductase inhibitors (statins) are a commonly prescribed class of medication for the treatment of hyperlipidemia and coronary artery disease. This class of medication has several proven benefits, including reduction of mortality related to coronary artery disease. A major consideration when prescribing these drugs are the potential for adverse effects, mainly myalgias, myopathy, and hepatotoxicity. In this article, we summarize current data on statin-associated hepatotoxicity and highlight that the risk of clinically significant idiosyncratic drug-induced liver injury is actually quite small. We also review preclinical data suggesting potential hepatoprotective effects of statin therapy.

No professional society has created guidelines to aid clinicians in the management of analgesics in the setting of hepatic injury. Acetaminophen overdose is the most common cause of acute liver failure in the United States. In the setting of acetaminophen toxicity, N-acetylcysteine remains the standard of care. Other analgesics including nonsteroidal antiinflammatory drugs, opiates, tricyclic antidepressants, and anticonvulsants rarely cause liver injury.

Although many risk factors for developing drug-induced liver injury (DILI) have been identified and more than 1000 medications and herbal and dietary supplements are known to cause liver dysfunction, idiosyncratic drug reactions remain unpredictable and erratic. Varying effects of individual drugs on the event cascade and patient genetic polymorphisms lead to different clinical presentations. Mechanisms and causality scales have been developed to guide the clinician in diagnosis, and several databases and registries are available for reference and reporting. We identify and summarize the resources available to clinicians to help diagnose, manage, and report DILI and to identify hepatotoxic drugs.

The use of herbal and dietary supplements (HDS) is increasing in the United States and worldwide. Its significant association with liver injury has become a concern, particularly because rates of hepatotoxicity caused by HDS are increasing. There are variety of HDS available, ranging from multi-ingredient substances, to anabolic steroids for bodybuilding purposes, to individual ingredients for purposes of supplementing a diet. This article reviews the impact of liver injury cause by HDS and explores the hepatotoxic potential of such products and their individual ingredients.

CLINICS IN LIVER DISEASE

Preface

A Focus on Drug-Induced Liver Injury

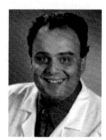

Pierre M. Gholam, MD, FAASLD
Editor

Drug-induced liver injury (DILI) is a clinically relevant, costly, and potentially catastrophic condition that affects persons in diverse settings of care. As indications for pharmacotherapy expand with the development of new drugs, so also does the potential for DILI in a greater number of people. The expansion of access to health care, including prescription drug coverage, in the United States may put more persons at risk for DILI. Though not well studied, it appears that recognition of patterns of injury consistent with DILI may not be optimal in primary care and even a more specialized setting. This knowledge gap creates an educational opportunity on which this issue of *Clinics in Liver Disease* focuses.

The reader is well introduced to the epidemiology of this global condition in both the general population and specific subsets. Host and environmental susceptibility are extensively covered. An entire article is dedicated to our growing understanding of the genetic underpinnings of DILI as well as the limitations of our current knowledge in this area. Illustrations of current and potential applications of genetic testing in DILI are also provided.

A comprehensive overview of our established methods of DILI causality assessment, including the Roussel Uclaf Causality Assessment Method, the Maria and Victorino Scale, and the Naranjo Adverse Drug Reactions Probability Scale, highlights the assets and limitations offered and introduces the reader to the DILI Network Structured Expert Opinion methodology and how it may help further our ability to better establish causality while raising issues of scalability. Clinicians will be well served to review an article dedicated to common patterns of injury and their potential corresponding offending agents.

The DILI-sim Initiative, a public-private partnership using Quantitative Systems Toxicology to build a model that may predict liver safety liabilities during drug development, provides mechanistic insights, predicts susceptible populations, and is

Clin Liver Dis 24 (2020) xiii–xiv
https://doi.org/10.1016/j.cld.2019.10.001
1089-3261/20/© 2019 Published by Elsevier Inc.

highlighted as a novel development that may enable a more refined approach to all these challenging issues.

No comprehensive review of DILI is complete without a dedicated histology article. Patterns of injury and other critical information, including prognosis, which a liver biopsy provides, are reviewed. Highly clinically relevant illustrations of these patterns of injury are provided and summarized in a table that both the nonspecialist and the consultant will find very useful.

No manifestation of DILI is more severe or dramatic than acute liver failure (ALF), which carries a high-mortality toll in the absence of the option of liver transplantation. The management of acetaminophen-induced ALF is expanded on. Importantly, the psychosocial liabilities of graft failure associated with ALF are presented. Of course, clinicians also face a dilemma in prescribing drugs known to have potential hepatotoxicity to persons with chronic liver disease. Our current understanding of this issue, which translates to clinical practice, is summarized.

Statins are arguably the most commonly prescribed pharmacologic agents in the United States and possibly worldwide. Not surprisingly, the issue of possible DILI secondary to statins comes up very frequently in a busy hepatology consultant's practice and affects a broad spectrum of prescribers and patients. This very relevant issue is explored with emphasis on not only the remarkable liver safety of these drugs in the general population but also their possible protective role in the setting of liver disease.

The last articles of this issue deliberately focus on agents that have come to occupy a disproportionate role in the cause of DILI in today's society. The uses and misuses of analgesics, including narcotics, are well documented, and insights into the potential DILI liabilities of these drugs are offered. Agents used for analgesia purposes that are covered include tricyclic antidepressants and anticonvulsants and also ubiquitously used nonsteroidal anti-inflammatory drugs, acetaminophen, and opioids.

We hope that this special DILI issue of *Clinics in Liver Disease* will be of use to both the busy clinician and the consultant. Ample references are provided at the end of each article to those interested in a deeper dive into any specific topic that the scope of this publication was unable to accommodate. A future that may include a more extensive use of personalized medicine may refine our decision-making process when drugs are prescribed and positively impact the significant toll of DILI in the general population.

Pierre M. Gholam, MD, FAASLD
Case Western Reserve University
School of Medicine
Liver Center of Excellence
University Hospitals Cleveland Medical Center
11100 Euclid Avenue
Cleveland, OH 44106, USA

E-mail address:
Pierre.gholam@case.edu

Epidemiology, Predisposing Factors, and Outcomes of Drug-Induced Liver Injury

Einar S. Björnsson, MD, PhD

KEYWORDS

- Drug-induced liver injury • Risk factors • Epidemiology • Prognosis

KEY POINTS

- The incidence of drug-induced liver injury (DILI) has in population-based studies been reported from 2.7 to 19 per 100,000 inhabitants a year.
- It is very difficult to predict the risk of developing DILI in the individual patient, but age and gender-related risks exist for certain drugs.
- Drug-induced jaundice is associated with a 10% to 50% risk of mortality based on the drug leading to liver injury.
- The prognosis for patients with acute liver failure due to *idiosyncratic* hepatotoxicity, is usually poor, with approximately 20% to 50% transplant-free survival.

INTRODUCTION

Drug-induced liver injury (DILI) is a potential complication of many drugs.[1–3] As the liver plays a central role in the metabolism of most drugs, this is not surprising. DILI is a not uncommon clinical entity and is an important differential diagnosis in patients with recent onset of elevated liver tests and normal hepatobiliary imaging. DILI is probably the most difficult to diagnose among known liver disorders, as it lacks a gold standard for confirmation. *Idiosyncratic* DILI is a major health concern in particular for patients who develop jaundice. Drug-induced jaundice carries a significant risk for liver failure with associated mortality and need for liver transplantation.

DILI has attracted increasing interest among researchers in recent years, as new therapies such as immunomodulatory therapies for inflammatory conditions and different malignancies have been shown to be associated with DILI. It is therefore a major concern for regulatory authorities supposed to protect safety of the users of

Disclosures: Declaration of personal and funding interests: The author has no conflicts of interests.

Department of Internal Medicine, Faculty of Medicine, Division of Gastroenterology and Hepatology, The National University Hospital of Iceland, University of Iceland, Hringbraut, Reykjavík 101, Iceland
E-mail address: einarsb@landspitali.is

Clin Liver Dis 24 (2020) 1–10
https://doi.org/10.1016/j.cld.2019.08.002

drugs as well as for the pharmaceutical industry. DILI is one of the most common reasons for termination of drug development of otherwise promising therapeutic agents after preclinical studies. DILI is an important drug safety issue and has become one of the major reasons of withdrawal of drugs shortly after being put onto the market. Moreover, DILI is the most common cause of acute liver failure (ALF) both in the United States and Europe.

In recent years, a few series with a large number of patients with DILI have been published.[1–3] Traditionally, DILI has been divided into intrinsic or dose-dependent liver injury, the best example being acetaminophen, and *idiosyncratic* thought to be independent of dose. However, recent studies have demonstrated that also *idiosyncratic* type of DILI or unpredictable liver injury related to drugs also has an important dose-dependent component.[4] The pathogenesis of DILI is largely unknown, and which patients are at risk is mostly unclear. Recent studies have led to an improved understanding of the pathogenesis. Certain HLA associations have been shown to be the major determinants of liver injury due to certain drugs[5,6] and other non-HLA genetic risk factors have recently been identified.[6,7]

Once DILI is suspected in a patient with new-onset liver disease, prompt cessation of drug(s) implicated is usually the first step in the management of DILI. It is obviously of crucial importance to assess the severity of the liver injury and symptomatic patients with jaundice and/or encephalopathy and/or coagulopathy should be hospitalized. Some of these patients will be in the need of a liver transplant that may be a life-saving procedure.

EPIDEMIOLOGY OF DRUG-INDUCED LIVER INJURY

Epidemiologic research on the risk of DILI took off in the early 1990s.[8–12] These studies were based on access to the General Practice Research Database (GPRD) in the United Kingdom. Before that, many commonly administered drugs were implicated in hepatotoxicity, but information was almost only available as case reports and spontaneous adverse drug reporting to national authorities.

Incidence

In the general population

There are very limited data reflecting the true incidence of DILI. Except within clinical trials, which can give reliable information about development of liver tests, there is great uncertainty on the occurrence of DILI associated with the clinical use of drugs. A few retrospective studies have tried to assess the incidence of DILI. A case control study in a large population in the GPRD, based on computer search identifying patients referred to a consultant or hospitalized for liver disease was perhaps the first study trying to analyze the incidence of DILI.[13] Crude incidence rates of DILIs in the United Kingdom were found to be 2.4 per 100,000 per year.[13] Remarkably similar incidence rates of 2.3 per 100,000 were demonstrated among outpatients in a university hospital clinic in Sweden.[14] A prospective nationwide study of DILI was undertaken recently in a university hospital over a 2-year period in in South Korea.[15] Hospitalization rates for DILI were used to extrapolate DILI, which was found to be 12 per 100,000 a year.[15] Herbal and dietary supplements (HDS) were the predominant causes of liver injury.[15] Similarly in other countries in Asia, such as Singapore, China, Japan, and India, herbal and traditional medicines are major reason for DILI.[16–21] Antituberculosis drugs are also a leading etiology of DILI in both India and China.[18,19]

Incidence rates obtained in retrospective surveys are likely to be an underestimation of the real incidence. This can be explained by the well-known underreporting of adverse reactions, difficulties to find these cases in medical record registries, due to the lack of uniform diagnoses, and difficulties to perform causality assessment in a retrospective study.

The first population-based study on liver injury associated with drugs was performed in a city in the north of France.[22] The French researchers did a careful prospective survey of DILIs aimed to assess the incidence and the seriousness of DILIs in a defined population.[22] All new cases of symptomatic DILIs were collected by physicians in a prospective fashion. The incidence of DILI was found to be 13.9 per 100,000 inhabitants.[22] A total of 12% required hospitalization and 6% died. Extrapolating these results to the whole general population in France, more than 8000 cases could occur in France per year leading to approximately 500 deaths. Taking into consideration the spontaneous reporting to the French Regulatory authorities, DILIs were at least 16 times more frequent than those obtained by spontaneous reporting. In a recent study undertaken in the total population of Iceland, patients with DILI were identified giving a crude annual incidence rate of 19.1 cases per 100,000 inhabitants.[23] Thus, the incidence of DILI in the general population of Iceland was found to be the highest reported to date. Amoxicillin-clavulanate was the most commonly implicated agent and detected in a higher proportion among hospitalized patients than outpatients. The highest risk of hepatotoxicity was found among users of azathioprine and infliximab.[23] The first prospective and population-based study performed in the United States was undertaken in Delaware, with a population of approximately 930,000.[24] The annual incidence was found to be 2.7 per 100,000 inhabitants and as in other prospective and retrospective DILI studies, antibiotics were the predominant drug class associated with DILI (36%), but a higher proportion of HDS than in other studies, in 43% of cases.[24] The incidence reported in the United States was lower than in other prospective population-based DILI studies,[22,25] but similar to previous retrospective studies.[13,14] Why the US study found a lower incidence than observed in Europe is unclear. The criteria for DILI were different, for example, in the French study,[22] the alanine aminotransferase (ALT) elevation threshold was only twofold and in the Icelandic study[23] threefold, but in the US study at least a fivefold increase in ALT to reach a threshold for DILI.[24] The study was also limited to gastroenterologists and hepatologists in contrast to previous prospective studies,[22,23] and the primary and the senior authors were not a part of the recruiting team.[24]

Among hospitalized patients and in patients with jaundice

In a study from Switzerland, of 4209 cases at risk of DILI among medical inpatients, the DILI prevalence at admission amounted to 0.7%.[26] The overall incidence of DILI during hospitalization was 1.4% but liver injury was not mentioned among diagnoses or in the discharge letter in more than half of the cases.[26] In consecutive patients hospitalized in the United Kingdom, evaluated by laboratory signals, 13 (8.8%) DILI cases were observed of 147 patients with liver enzyme elevations among 1964 admissions, giving an incidence of 0.7% of inpatients.[27] A similar tendency was observed in patients with drug-associated liver enzyme abnormalities seen in patients under the care of a health maintenance organization in the United States.[28] Physicians, frequently discontinued the suspected drugs but did not ascribe the liver test abnormalities to drugs in the medical records.[28] These studies are for many reasons likely to be an underestimation of DILI in hospitalized patients.

Acute hepatic injury due to drugs has been reported to occur in between 2% and 10% of patients hospitalized for jaundice. In Sweden, 2% to 3% of patients hospitalized for jaundice were considered to be due to DILI.[29] In a recent study from the United

States, acute liver disease as a result of nonalcoholic etiologies was caused by DILI in 4% of cases with jaundice.[30]

Drug-induced liver injury among patients with acute liver failure

Drugs are the most common cause of fulminant hepatic failure in the United States, Europe, and Japan.[25,31–33] Acetaminophen is the single most common cause of ALF in the Western world[25,31,33] and *idiosyncratic* drug reactions were the presumptive causes in 13% to 17% of cases of ALF in the United States and Sweden.[25,31,33] Furthermore, liver transplantation for drug hepatotoxicity accounted for 15% of liver transplants for ALF in the United States.[34] A recent study, also from the United States on the incidence of drug-induced ALF, from the Kaiser Permanente health care system showed acetaminophen to be the most common cause of ALF.[35] Although uncommon, *idiosyncratic* drug-induced ALF was associated with severe outcomes, with 30% mortality rate and/or need for liver transplantation.[35] HDSs were the most common cause of drug-induced ALF followed by antimicrobials.[35]

Predisposing Factors

Genetic predisposition is discussed in detail in Camilla Stephens and Raúl J. Andrade's article, "Genetic Predisposition to Drug-Induced Liver Injury," elsewhere in this issue, so this article focuses on nongenetic risk factors.

Age and Gender

A relationship was observed between the incidence of DILI and higher age in the prospective DILI study from Iceland.[23] However, that does not necessarily imply a causal relationship and might reflect an increased number of drugs prescribed in older people. The phenotype of DILI seems to be affected by advanced age, as cholestatic type of DILI seems to be more common in patients older than 60 years.[36] In contrast, hepatocellular type of DILI is more common in younger patients, but the reason for this is unclear.[14,36] It is not clear why cholestatic type of DILI is more common in the elderly. This might be influenced by impaired renal function, decreased hepatic blood flow, and decreased hepatic mass with advanced age.[37,38] Age seems to be a risk factor for DILI associated with the use of specific drugs. The risk of DILI has been shown to increase with advanced age for drugs such as nitrofurantoin,[39] isoniazid,[40] flucloxacillin,[41] and amoxicillin-clavulanate.[42] On the other hand, younger age (children <10 years) is a risk factor for valproic acid.[43]

In general, female and male individuals seem to have similar risk of developing liver injury from drugs.[1–3,14,36] However, female patients seem to have an increased risk of developing liver injury from certain drugs such as nitrofurantoin,[39] flucloxacillin,[41] and diclofenac.[44] Zimmerman[45] pointed out that drug-induced autoimmune hepatitis seems to occur almost exclusively in women, which was later confirmed in other studies.[46–48] Hepatocellular type of DILI has been shown to occur more commonly in female than male individuals.[3,36] The severity of DILI has been associated with female sex and in the Spanish Registry.[36] The vast majority (90%) of patients with fulminant hepatic failure from DILI were women, and female sex was an independent risk factor for ALF from drugs.[36] Also 77% of patients with ALF in the United States were women.[25]

Race

It is unclear if the risk for DILI is associated with ethnicity, and this has not been well documented. "Chronicity," defined as elevated liver tests 6 months after presentation of DILI, was more common in African American individuals than in other races.[49] Asian race was also an independent risk factor for the need for liver transplantation from DILI.[49] The reason for these findings is unclear and has not been confirmed in other studies. A recent study drug-induced liver injury network (DILIN) group found that African American individuals had higher rates of liver-related death and liver transplantation at 6 months compared with Caucasians.[50]

Concomitant Disorders

There are few data to suggest that comorbidities have major impact on the risk of developing DILI. Diabetes mellitus (DM) does not seem to increase the risk for DILI in general.[1–3] DM and obesity have been shown to be risk factors for methotrexate-induced liver injury.[51,52] DM has also been associated with increased risk of mortality in patients with DILI.[3,53] Furthermore, DM was associated with increased risk of chronic DILI in patients followed within the Spanish Hepatotoxicity Registry.[54]

It is somewhat controversial whether chronic liver disease increases the risk of developing DILI.[55,56] In a landmark paper, Chalasani and colleagues[57] demonstrated that patients with elevated liver tests at baseline did not have an increased risk of hepatotoxicity from statins. Others have confirmed these observations in patients with hepatitis C and nonalcoholic fatty liver disease.[58,59]

In some studies, patients with chronic viral hepatitis, have been reported to be at an increased risk of hepatotoxicity due to antituberculosis drugs.[60–63] Other studies have not shown this increased risk in patients with chronic liver disease.[64–66] Coinfection with human immunodeficiency virus and hepatitis C virus was found to increase the risk of hepatoxicity.[67] Other studies have also found liver injury associated with the use of antiretroviral drugs to be higher in patients coinfected with hepatitis B and C.[68–73] Causality assessment of the potential DILI has not been well reported in these studies, and exclusion of competing etiologies has not been well described. Confounding factors exist that make the interpretation of these results difficult. Spontaneous fluctuations in viral loads are common in both hepatitis C[74,75] and hepatitis B,[76,77] which has to be taken into consideration when assessing the etiology of elevated liver tests in these patients. Control groups of patients with viral hepatitis not on the drugs have been lacking in these studies.

Although patients with chronic liver disease do not in general have an increased risk of developing DILI, the consequences of a DILI in these patients might be more severe.[45] In a recent article from the DILIN network, mortality from DILI was significantly higher in patients with preexisting liver disease.[53]

Outcomes of Drug-Induced Liver Injury

The vast majority of patients with DILI recover clinically and biochemically when the implicated agent has been discontinued.[1–3] Patients recruited in population-based cohorts have generally less severe liver injury at baseline[22–24] as compared with patients seen at referral centers,[1,3,45] and the latter patient category has worse prognosis.

Hyman Zimmerman,[45] a pioneer researcher in the field of DILI, observed that the combination of hepatocellular injury and jaundice induced by a drug was associated with a poor prognosis with a fatality rate of 10% to 50% for the different drugs involved (so called Hy's rule). This has been confirmed in other studies.[1–3] Once a patient develops jaundice due to drugs, what are the most important determinants of prognosis? The prognosis for patients with ALF due to *idiosyncratic* hepatotoxicity, is usually poor, with approximately 20% to 50% transplant-free survival.[31] Prognosis is generally more favorable in paracetamol-induced ALF with 60% to 80% reported transplant-free survival.[31]

Researchers from the Spanish DILI developed a model for predicting ALF in patients with DILI.[78] Use of a new R value (nR) using either ALT or aspartate aminotransferase, whichever is highest, improved ALF prediction.[78] Better prediction for fatality with nR Hy's law was recently confirmed.[79]

REFERENCES

1. Andrade RJ, Lucena MI, Fernandez MC, et al. Drug-induced liver injury: an analysis of 461 incidences submitted to the Spanish registry over a 10-year period. Gastroenterology 2005;129:512–21.
2. Bjornsson E, Olsson R. Outcome and prognostic markers in severe drug-induced liver disease. Hepatology 2005;42:481–9.
3. Chalasani N, Fontana RJ, Bonkovsky HL, et al. Causes, clinical features, and outcomes from a prospective study of drug-induced liver injury in the United States. Gastroenterology 2008;135:1924–34.
4. Lammert C, Einarsson S, Saha C, et al. Relationship between daily dose of oral medications and idiosyncratic drug-induced liver injury: search for signals. Hepatology 2008;47:2003–9.
5. Daly AK, Donaldson PT, Bhatnagar P, et al. HLA-B*5701 genotype is a major determinant of drug-induced liver injury due to flucloxacillin. Nat Genet 2009; 41:816–9.
6. Nicoletti P, Aithal GP, Bjornsson ES, et al. Association of liver injury from specific drugs, or groups of drugs, with polymorphisms in HLA and other genes in a genome-wide association study. Gastroenterology 2017;152:1078–89.
7. Cirulli ET, Nicoletti P, Abramson K, et al. Identification of a PTPN22 missense variant as a general genetic risk factor for drug-induced liver injury. Gastroenterology 2019. https://doi.org/10.1053/j.gastro.2019.01.034.
8. Jick H, Derby LE, García Rodríguez LA, et al. Liver disease associated with diclofenac, naproxen and piroxicam. Pharmacotherapy 1992;12:207–12.
9. Derby LE, Jick H, Henry DA, et al. Cholestatic hepatitis associated with flucloxacillin. Med J Aust 1993;158(9):596–600.
10. Derby LE, Gutthann SP, Jick H, et al. Liver disorders in patients receiving chlorpromazine or isoniazid. Pharmacotherapy 1993;13:353–8.
11. Garcia Rodriguez LA, Stricker BH, Zimmerman HJ. Risk of acute liver injury associated with the combination of amoxicillin and clavulanic acid. Arch Intern Med 1996;156:1327–32.
12. Garcia Rodriguez LA, Williams R, Derby LE, et al. Acute liver injury associated with nonsteroidal anti-in flammatory drugs and the role of risk factors. Arch Intern Med 1994;154:311–6.
13. de Abajo FJ, Montero D, Madurga M, et al. Acute and clinically relevant drug-induced liver injury: a population based case-control study. Br J Clin Pharmacol 2004;58:71–80.
14. De Valle MB, Av Klinteberg V, Alem N, et al. Drug-induced liver injury in a Swedish University hospital out-patient hepatology clinic. Aliment Pharmacol Ther 2006; 24:1187–95.
15. Suk KT, Kim DJ, Kim CH, et al. A prospective nationwide study of drug-induced liver injury in Korea. Am J Gastroenterol 2012;107:1380–7.
16. Wai CT, Tan BH, Chan CL, et al. Drug-induced liver injury at an Asian center: a prospective study. Liver Int 2007;27:465–74.
17. Takikawa H, Murata Y, Horiike N, et al. Drug-induced liver injury in Japan: an analysis of 1676 cases between 1997 and 2006. Hepatol Res 2009;39:427–31.

18. Devarbhavi H, Dierkhising R, Kremers WK, et al. Single-center experience with drug-induced liver injury from India: causes, outcome, prognosis and predictors of mortality. Am J Gastroenterol 2010;105:2396–404.

19. Zhou Y, Yang L, Liao Z, et al. Epidemiology of drug-induced liver injury in China: a systematic analysis of the Chinese literature including 21,789 patients. Eur J Gastroenterol Hepatol 2013;25:825–9.

20. Devarbhavi H, Patil M, Reddy VV, et al. Drug induced acute liver failure in children and adults: results of a single-centre study of 128 patients. Liver Int 2017;38: 1322–9.

21. Devarbhavi H. Ayurvedic and herbal medicine-induced liver injury: it is time to wake up and take notice. Indian J Gastroenterol 2018;37:5–7.

22. Sgro C, Clinard F, Ouazir K, et al. Incidence of drug-induced hepatic injuries: a French population-based study. Hepatology 2002;36:451–5.

23. Bjornsson ES, Bergmann OM, Bjornsson HK, et al. Incidence, presentation and outcomes in patients with drug-induced liver injury in the general population of Iceland. Gastroenterology 2013;144:1419–25.

24. Vega M, Verma M, Beswick D, et al. The incidence of drug- and herbal and dietary supplement-induced liver injury: preliminary findings from gastroenterologist-based surveillance in the population of the state of Delaware. Drug Saf 2017;40: 783–7.

25. Reuben A, Koch DG, Lee WM. Drug-induced acute liver failure: results of a U.S. multicenter, prospective study. Hepatology 2010;52:2065–76.

26. Meier Y, Cavallaro M, Roos M, et al. Incidence of drug-induced liver injury in medical inpatients. Eur J Clin Pharmacol 2005;61:135–43.

27. Bagheri H, Michel F, Lapeyre-Mestre M, et al. Detection and incidence of drug-induced liver injuries in hospital: a prospective analysis from laboratory signals. Br J Clin Pharmacol 2000;50:479–84.

28. Duh MS, Walker AM, Kronlund KH Jr. Descriptive epidemiology of acute liver enzyme abnormalities in the general population of central Massachusetts. Pharmacoepidemiol Drug Saf 1999;8:275–83.

29. Björnsson E, Ismael S, Nejdet S, et al. Severe jaundice in Sweden in the new millennium: causes, investigations, treatment and prognosis. Scand J Gastroenterol 2003;38:86–94.

30. Vuppalanchi R, Liangpunsakul S, Chalasani N. Etiology of new-onset jaundice: how often is it caused by idiosyncratic drug-induced liver injury in the United States. Am J Gastroenterol 2006;101:1–5.

31. Ostapowicz G, Fontana RJ, Schiodt FV, et al. U.S. Acute Liver Failure Study Group. Results of a prospective study of acute liver failure at 17 tertiary care centers in the United States. Ann Intern Med 2002;137:947–54.

32. Ohmori S, Shiraki K, Inoue H, et al. Clinical characteristics and prognostic indicators of drug-induced fulminant hepatic failure. Hepatogastroenterology 2003;50: 1531–4.

33. Wei G, Bergquist A, Broome U, et al. Acute liver failure in Sweden: etiology and outcome. J Intern Med 2007;262:392–401.

34. Russo MW, Galanko JA, Shrestha R, et al. Liver transplantation for acute liver failure from drug induced liver injury in the United States. Liver Transpl 2004;10: 1018–23.

35. Goldberg DS, Forde KA, Carbonari DM, et al. Population-representative incidence of drug-induced acute liver failure based on an analysis of an integrated health care system. Gastroenterology 2015;148:1353–61.

36. Lucena MI, Andrade RJ, Kaplowitz N, et al. Phenotypic characterization of idiosyncratic drug-induced liver injury: the influence of age and gender. Hepatology 2009;49:2001–9.

37. Mitchell SJ, Hilmer SN. Drug-induced liver injury in older adults. Ther Adv Drug Saf 2010;1:65–77.

38. Ort Ortega-Alonso A, Stephens C, Lucena MI, et al. Case characterization, clinical features and risk factors in drug-induced liver injury. Int J Mol Sci 2016;17(5) [pii:E714].

39. Holmberg L, Boman G, Böttiger LE, et al. Adverse reactions to nitrofurantoin. Analysis of 921 reports. Am J Med 1980;69:733–8.

40. Fountain FF, Tolley E, Chrisman CR, et al. Isoniazid hepatotoxicity associated with treatment of latent tuberculosis infection: a 7-year evaluation from a public health tuberculosis clinic. Chest 2005;128:116–23.

41. Olsson R, Wiholm BE, Sand C, et al. Liver damage from flucloxacillin, cloxacillin and dicloxacillin. J Hepatol 1992;15(1–2):154–61.

42. Lucena MI, Andrade RJ, Fernandez MC, et al. Determinants of the clinical expression of amoxicillin-clavulanate hepatotoxicity: a prospective series from Spain. Hepatology 2006;44:850–6.

43. Dreifuss FE, Santilli N, Langer DH, et al. Valproic acid hepatic fatalities: a retrospective review. Neurology 1987;37(3):379–85.

44. Banks AT, Zimmerman HJ, Ishak KG, et al. Diclofenac-associated hepatotoxicity: analysis of 180 cases reported to the Food and Drug Administration as adverse reactions. Hepatology 1995;22(3):820–7.

45. Zimmerman HJ. Hepatotoxicity: the adverse effects of drugs and other chemicals on the liver. 2nd edition. Philadelphia: Lippincott; 1999. p. 603–5.

46. Björnsson E, Talwalkar J, Treeprasertsuk S, et al. Drug-induced autoimmune hepatitis: clinical characteristics and prognosis. Hepatology 2010;51:2040–8.

47. Björnsson ES, Gunnarsson BI, Gröndal G, et al. The risk of drug-induced liver injury from Tumor Necrosis Factor (TNF)-alpha-antagonists. Clin Gastroenterol Hepatol 2015;13:602–8.

48. Björnsson E, Bergmann O, Jonasson JG, et al. Drug-induced autoimmune hepatitis: response to corticosteroids and lack of relapse after cessation of steroids. Clin Gastroenterol Hepatol 2017;15:1635–6.

49. Fontana RJ, Hayashi PH, Gu J, et al. Idiosyncratic drug-induced liver injury is associated with substantial morbidity and mortality within 6 months from onset. Gastroenterology 2014;147:96–108.

50. Chalasani N, Reddy K, Fontana RJ, et al. Idiosyncratic drug induced liver injury in African-Americans is associated with greater morbidity and mortality compared to Caucasians. Am J Gastroenterol 2017;112:1382–8.

51. Malatjalian DA, Ross JB, Williams CN, et al. Methotrexate hepatotoxicity in psoriatics: report of 104 patients from Nova Scotia, with analysis of risks from obesity, diabetes and alcohol consumption during long term follow-up. Can J Gastroenterol 1996;10:369–75.

52. Rosenberg P, Urwitz H, Johannesson A, et al. Psoriasis patients with diabetes type 2 are at high risk of developing liver fibrosis during methotrexate treatment. J Hepatol 2007;46:1111–8.

53. Chalasani N, Bonkovsky HL, Fontana R, et al. Features and outcomes of 899 patients with drug-induced liver injury: the DILIN prospective study. Gastroenterology 2015;148:1340–52.

54. Medina-Caliz I, Robles-Diaz M, Garcia-Muñoz B, et al. Definition and risk factors for chronicity following acute idiosyncratic drug-induced liver injury. J Hepatol 2016 Sep;65(3):532–42.

55. Lewis JH. The rational use of potentially hepatotoxic medications in patients with underlying liver disease. Expert Opin Drug Saf 2002;1:159–72.

56. Russo MW, Watkins PB. Are patients with elevated liver tests at increased risk of drug-induced liver injury? Gastroenterology 2004;126:1477–80.

57. Chalasani N, Aljadhey H, Kesterson J, et al. Patients with elevated liver enzymes are not at higher risk for statin hepatotoxicity. Gastroenterology 2004;126:1287–92.

58. Lewis JH, Mortensen ME, Zweig S, et al. Efficacy and safety of high-dose pravastatin in hypercholesterolemic patients with well-compensated chronic liver disease: results of a prospective, randomized, double-blind, placebo-controlled, multicenter trial. Hepatology 2007;46:1453–63.

59. Ekstedt M, Franzen LE, Mathiesen UL, et al. Statins in non-alcoholic fatty liver disease and chronically elevated liver enzymes: a histopathological follow-up study. J Hepatol 2007;47:135–41.

60. Wong WM, Wu PC, Yuen MF, et al. Antituberculosis drug-related liver dysfunction in chronic hepatitis B infection. Hepatology 2000;31:201–6.

61. Lee BH, Koh WJ, Choi MS, et al. Inactive hepatitis B surface antigen carrier state and hepatotoxicity during antituberculosis chemotherapy. Chest 2005;127:1304–11.

62. Patel PA, Voigt MD. Prevalence and interaction of hepatitis B and latent tuberculosis in Vietnamese immigrants to the United States. Am J Gastroenterol 2002;97:1198–203.

63. Wang JY, Liu CH, Hu FC, et al. Risk factors of hepatitis during anti-tuberculous treatment and implications of hepatitis virus load. J Infect 2011;62:448–55.

64. Hwang SJ, Wu JC, Lee CN, et al. A prospective clinical study of isoniazid-rifampicin-pyrazinamide-induced liver injury in an area endemic for hepatitis B. J Gastroenterol Hepatol 1997;12:87–91.

65. Shu CC, Lee CH, Lee MC, et al. Hepatotoxicity due to first-line anti-tuberculosis drugs: a five-year experience in a Taiwan medical centre. Int J Tuberc Lung Dis 2013;17:934–9.

66. Liu YM, Cheng YJ, Li YL, et al. Antituberculosis treatment and hepatotoxicity in patients with chronic viral hepatitis. Lung 2014;192:205–10.

67. Ungo JR, Jones D, Ashkin D, et al. Antituberculosis drug-induced hepatotoxicity. The role of hepatitis C virus and the human immunodeficiency virus. Am J Respir Crit Care Med 1998;157:1871–6.

68. den Brinker M, Wit FW, Wertheim-van Dillen PM, et al. Hepatitis B and C virus co-infection and the risk for hepatotoxicity of highly active antiretroviral therapy in HIV-1 infection. AIDS 2000;14:2895–902.

69. Bonfanti P, Landonio S, Ricci E, et al. Risk factors for hepato-toxicity in patients treated with highly active antiretroviral therapy. J Acquir Immune Defic Syndr 2001;27:316–8.

70. Aceti A, Pasquazzi C, Zechini B, et al. Hepatotoxicity development during antiretroviral therapy containing protease inhibitors in patients with HIV: the role of hepatitis B and C virus infection. J Acquir Immune Defic Syndr 2002;29(1):41–8.

71. Bonacini M. Liver injury during highly active antiretroviral therapy: the effect of hepatitis C coinfection. Clin Infect Dis 2004;38(Suppl 2):S104–8.

72. Kramer JR, Giordano TP, Souchek J, et al. Hepatitis C coinfection increases the risk of fulminant hepatic failure in patients with HIV in the HAART era. J Hepatol 2005;42:309–14.
73. Sulkowski MS, Thomas DL, Mehta SH, et al. Hepatotoxicity associated with nevirapine or efavirenz-containing antiretroviral therapy: role of hepatitis C and B infections. Hepatology 2002;35:182–9.
74. Arase Y, Ikeda K, Chayama K, et al. Fluctuation patterns of HCV-RNA serum level in patients with chronic hepatitis C. J Gastroenterol 2000;35:221–5.
75. ItoH, Yoshioka K, Ukai K, et al. The fluctuation of viral load and serum alanine aminotransferase levels in chronic hepatitis C. Hepatol Res 2004;30:11–7.
76. Brunetto MR, Oliveri F, Coco B, et al. Outcome of anti-HBe positive chronic hepatitis B in alpha-interferon treated and un- treated patients: a long term cohort study. J Hepatol 2002;36:263–70.
77. Jain MK, Parekh NK, Hester J, et al. Aminotransferase elevation in HIV/hepatitis B virus co-infected patients treated with two active hepatitis B virus drugs. AIDS Patient Care STDS 2006;20:817–22.
78. Robles–Diaz M, Lucena MI, Kaplowitz N, et al. Use of Hy's law and a new composite algorithm to predict acute liver failure in patients with drug-induced liver injury. Gastroenterology 2014;147:109–18.e5.
79. Hayashi PH, Rockey DC, Fontana RJ, et al. Death and liver transplantation within 2 years of onset of drug-induced liver injury. Hepatology 2017;66:1275–85.

Genetic Predisposition to Drug-Induced Liver Injury

Camilla Stephens, PhD[a,b], Raúl J. Andrade, MD, PhD[a,b,*]

KEYWORDS

- Candidate gene studies • Genome-wide association studies • Drug metabolism
- Pharmacogenetics • Pharmacogenomics • Human leukocyte antigen

KEY POINTS

- Genetic risk factors in drug-induced liver injury (DILI) support that the immune system is an integral component in DILI development.
- HLA risk alleles have low positive predictive value and therefore do not meet the threshold for clinical application in the form of pre-prescription genetic screening to prevent DILI.
- HLA risk alleles can support or refute a DILI diagnosis and provide guidance on the most likely causative agent in patients exposed to multiple drugs.
- HLA risk alleles can assist in distinguishing DILI with autoimmune features from idiopathic autoimmune hepatitis.

INTRODUCTION

Idiosyncratic drug-induced liver injury (which will be referred to simply as DILI throughout this review) is a rare, yet potentially life-threatening, form of adverse drug reaction. It is thought to occur through a combination of drug properties, host factors, and environmental conditions. Hence, DILI is not predictable from drug dosage and pharmacologic action, as is the case with intrinsic hepatotoxicity, as exemplified by acetaminophen overdose. The idiosyncratic nature of DILI has limited the development of functional animal research models and consequently slowed down the progress toward a complete understanding of the pathogenesis. Nevertheless, it is generally believed that DILI is a multifactorial condition with several

Disclosure: The authors have nothing to disclose.
Funding: This work was supported by grants of the Instituto de Salud Carlos III co-founded by Fondo Europeo de Desarrollo Regional - FEDER (contract numbers: PI16/01748 and PI18/00901). CIBERehd is funded by Instituto de Salud Carlos III.
[a] Unidad de Gestión Clínica de Aparato Digestivo, Instituto de Investigación Biomédica de Málaga-IBIMA, Hospital Universitario Virgen de la Victoria, Universidad de Málaga, Boulevard Louis Pasteur 32, Málaga, 29071 Spain; [b] Centro de Investigación Biomédica en Red de Enfermedades Hepáticas y Digestivas (CIBERehd), Spain
* Corresponding author. Facultad de Medicina, Universidad de Málaga, Boulevard Louis Pasteur 32, Málaga 29071, Spain.
E-mail address: andrade@uma.es

mechanisms and cellular pathways involved. The initial step of DILI is assumed to be hepatocyte exposure to some form of stress induced by the causative agent, with reactive metabolites formed during drug metabolism often playing a pivotal role. Genetic variations in the host that favor increased exposure to reactive metabolites (increased production and/or reduced detoxification/clearance) have therefore long been the focus of DILI genetic studies to identify variations that predispose an individual to DILI susceptibility.

In addition to drug metabolism, the immune system is also considered an important component in DILI development. Reactive metabolites can function as haptens that bind to endogenous proteins and subsequently form neoantigens, which, when presented on specific HLA molecules, may elicit an inappropriate immune response that contributes to perpetuation of liver damage. This theory is supported by findings of associations between specific human HLA alleles and increased risk of DILI, including with causative agents that normally do not manifest clinical signs of immunopathology.

Understanding the genetic basis for disease susceptibility has become an increasingly important target in biomedicine. Genetic studies in search for specific alleles that influence DILI susceptibility have been undertaken for decades, initially using candidate gene (CG) studies and more recently through genome-wide association (GWA) studies. Data on the functional significance of many polymorphisms in the targeted genes are emerging, which provides new insight into DILI on a cellular level. However, most genetic risk factors identified to date lack strong effect sizes. This is in line with the hypothesis of DILI being a multifactorial condition, but also restricts the use of these variations in the form of genetic testing in clinical practice.

CANDIDATE GENE STUDIES

The CG approach is the classic form of identifying genetic variations associated with clinical traits. It is relatively cheap and rapid to perform, but requires prior information on the disease mechanism to select genes and subsequent polymorphisms of interest. The CG studies in DILI have, to a large extent, focused on genes involved in drug metabolism, because polymorphisms in these genes can potentially change the concentration of drug metabolites through increased formation and/or decreased clearance in patients treated with standard medication doses. It has been estimated that polymorphisms in drug-metabolizing genes influence the clinical outcome in 20% to 25% of all drug therapies.[1] The biological function and considerable level of interindividual variations known to exist in genes involved in drug metabolism pathways therefore make them plausible targets for DILI susceptibility. Genetic variations identified through CG studies as involved in DILI susceptibility are outlined in **Table 1**.

Phase I (Bioactivation)

Reactive metabolites are formed during drug metabolism, usually through the initiation of cytochrome P450 (CYP450)-mediated reactions. Although reactive metabolites is not a prerequisite for DILI development because drugs unknown to form reactive metabolites also cause DILI, a study of 254 drugs found that drugs that are CYP450 substrates have a higher likelihood of causing DILI.[2] However, few reports on CYP variations strongly associated with increased DILI susceptibility are available (see **Table 1**). Earlier studies focusing on genetic variation in CYP2C8, CYP2C9, and CYP2C19 did not find any specific alleles being significantly associated with DILI.[3–5] Genetic variations linked to CYP2B6 have, however, been associated with increased risk of hepatotoxicity following ticlopidine in Japanese patients and efavirenz-based

Table 1
Genetic polymorphisms associated with drug-induced liver injury identified in candidate gene studies

Gene (Risk Allele or Genotype)	Causative Drug (Cohort Population)	Association (Odds Ratio)	Reference
CYP2B6, rs7254579 (C)	Ticlopidine (Japanese)	Risk (2.1)	Ariyoshi et al,[6] 2010
CYP2B6 (*6/*6)	Efavirenz-based HAART (African)	Risk (3.3)	Yimer et al,[7] 2012
CYP2A6*4	Valproic acid (Chinese)	Risk (2.5–20)	Zhao et al,[8] 2017
CYP2E1 (c1/c1)	Anti-TBC (Taiwanese)	Risk (2.5)	Huang et al,[9] 2003
UGT2B7 (*2)	Diclofenac (European)	Risk (7.7–8.5)	Daly et al,[4] 2007
UGT1A6 (various SNPs)	Tolcapone (European)	Risk (2.8)	Acuña et al,[12] 2002
NAT2 (slow acetylator)	Anti-TBC (Asian)	Risk (3.0–3.2)	Du et al,[13] 2013
NAT2 (slow acetylator)	Anti-TBC (White)	None	Du et al,[13] 2013
NAT2 (slow acetylator)	Anti-TBC (Asian)	Risk (3.0–6.4)	Zhang et al,[14] 2018
NAT2 (slow acetylator)	Anti-TBC (White)	Risk (2.0–2.3)	Zhang et al,[14] 2018
GSTM1/T1 (null)	Tacrine (European)	Risk (2.3)	Simon et al,[16] 2000
GSTM1/T1 (null)	Troglitazone (Japanese)	Risk (3.7)	Watanabe et al,[17] 2003
GSTM1/T1 (null)	Anti-TBC (Indian)	Risk (7.2)	Gupta et al,[18] 2013
GSTM1/T1 (null)	Various (European)	Risk (2.7–5.6)	Lucena et al,[19] 2008
ABCB1 rs1045642 (T)	Nevirapine (African)	Protection (0.3)	Haas et al,[23] 2006
ABCB1 rs1045642 (T)	Nevirapine (North American)	Protection (0.25)	Ritchie et al,[24] 2006
ABCB1 rs1045642 (T)	Nevirapine (African)	Protection (0.4)	Ciccacci et al,[25] 2010
ABCB1 rs2032582 (G)	Atorvastatin (Japanese)	Risk (2.6)	Fukunaga et al,[26] 2016
ABCC2 -24T	Diclofenac (European)	Risk (5.0–6.0)	Daly et al,[4] 2007

Abbreviations: HAART, highly active antiretroviral therapy; TBC, tuberculosis.

highly active antiretroviral therapy (HAART) in Ethiopian patients, although these findings have not been confirmed in independent cohorts.[6,7] The identified risk allele of the single-nucleotide polymorphism (SNP) associated with ticlopidine hepatotoxicity (rs7254579, C) was reported to increase CYP2B6 expression and may subsequently increase the level of reactive metabolites.[6] In contrast, the CYP2B6*6 risk allele for efavirenz-based HAART hepatotoxicity is associated with decreased CYP2B6 activity that could lead to a potential accumulation of the parent drug, which is consistent with pharmacokinetic findings for efavirenz in the study cohort.[7] This suggests that the parent drug may play a more important role than metabolites in efavirenz-induced hepatotoxicity. Chinese carriers of the CYP2A6*4 allele leading to a poor metabolizer phenotype have been found to be more prone to aminotransferase elevations after initiating valproic acid treatment. These patients also had higher serum concentration of the intermediate drug metabolites 4-ene-valproic acid and 2,4-diene-valproic acid, which are believed to be involved in valproic acid hepatotoxicity, although the exact role of CYP2A6 in valproate metabolism is not yet elucidated.[8]

The CYP2E1 gene has been the target of many pharmacogenetics studies on anti-tuberculosis (anti-TBC) treatments. Carriers homozygous for the CYP2E1 wild-type c1 allele was first associated with increased risk of DILI owing to anti-TBC drugs in Taiwanese patients. This genotype leads to higher CYP2E1 activity than genotypes including variant alleles, and may lead to increased level of hepatotoxic metabolites, particularly with isoniazid.[9] This result has since been replicated in various independent studies and a meta-analysis on 26 different studies found that the c1/c1 genotype was in fact associated with increased risk of anti-TBC hepatotoxicity, but with a relatively small effect size (odds ratio 1.3).[10] It should be pointed out that the studies included in this meta-analysis varied with regard to anti-TBC regimens and hepatotoxicity definition, with many studies including cases with mild transaminase elevations. Self-limiting drug-related events ("adaptations") are therefore likely to have been included in some of the studies, because anti-TBC regimens are well known to cause this form of clinically unimportant events. Furthermore, most of the study cohorts were Asian or South American, with limited representation of white patients.

Phase II (Detoxification)

Intermediate drug metabolites are detoxified through conjugation reactions catalyzed by phase II enzymes. One of the more important enzymes here is UDP-glucuronosyltransferase (UGT). The *UGT2B7*2* allele, has been associated with increased risk of diclofenac-induced liver injury, with the corresponding gene product hypothesized to have higher catalytic activity, and subsequent diclofenac hepatotoxicity potentially mediated through increased level of diclofenac acylglucuronide.[4] A recent study, however, found that the *UGT2B7*2* enzyme had 6-fold lower activity of diclofenac glucuronidation compared with the wild-type, *UGT2B7*1*. The same group hypothesized that the association between *UGT2B7*2* and increased risk of diclofenac hepatotoxicity might therefore stem from a shift to oxidative bioactivation leading to cytotoxic quinoneimine formation.[11] In addition, several SNPs located within *UGT1A*, particularly *UGT1A6* and *UGT1A7*, have been associated with tolcapone-induced transaminase elevations, potentially through decreased enzymatic activity. Because glucuronidation is the main pathway for tolcapone elimination, one can hypothesize that impaired clearance of tolcapone may contribute to hepatotoxicity.[12] However, the low cutoff point for transaminase elevations in this study, which did not reach the current threshold for clinically important DILI, could have contributed to inclusion of patients with non-DILI-related transaminase elevations.

N-Acetyltransferase 2 (NAT2) has been the focus of various anti-TBC hepatotoxicity studies over the last 2 decades. This enzyme is involved in various aspects of isoniazid metabolism, including both metabolite formation and detoxification. The presence of two copies of any of several mutant alleles of the *NAT2* gene is well known to provide a slow acetylation phenotype. Many CG studies to date have demonstrated that carriers of *NAT2* slow acetylator genotypes are overall more susceptible to hepatotoxicity induced by isoniazid-based anti-TBC regimens, as reflected in large meta-analyses. However stratified by ethnicity, Caucasians were found to have lower or no association, whereas associations with larger effect sizes were seen for Asians.[13,14] This could be due to genetic differences between different ethnicities, but also to the fact that limited studies on *NAT2* in anti-TBC hepatotoxicity have been performed using cohorts of European origin. Similar to the findings for *CYP2E1* polymorphisms, the effect size of the *NAT2* slow acetylator genotype is relatively small and many studies included small numbers of cases and/or cases with limited liver profile elevations not reaching clinical relevance. In contrast, a recent GWA study of 59 Indian patients with anti-TBC hepatotoxicity failed to detect any genome-wide significant associations for genotyped variants and imputed NAT2 acetylator status, compared with 220 controls. The complexity of anti-TBC treatments in terms of being multiple drug combinations may require higher study power, which was limited by the low number of study subjects, to determine significant associations.[15]

Glutathione-S-transferase (GST) *catalyzes* the conjugation of reduced glutathione to xenobiotic substrates, including intermediate drug metabolites, to facilitate cellular excretion. In addition to drug metabolism, GST is important in cellular protection against oxidative stress. Several GST isozymes are present in humans, but genetic DILI studies have focused mainly on *GSTT1* and *GSTM1*. Null variants are available for both *GSTT1* and *GSTM1*, whereby the entire gene is deleted leading to complete absence of enzyme activity. A number of studies have found that homozygous GSTM1/GSTT1 null carriers are more susceptible to DILI induced by tacrine,[16] troglitazone,[17] anti-TBC therapy,[18] and drugs in general,[19] although studies that did not find any association are also available.[20,21] It has been suggested that inconsistent results of disease risk associated with *GST* null variants could stem from variations in overexpression of other *GST* genes, such as *GSTM2*, to compensate for the presence of null alleles.[22]

Phase III (Clearance)

Genetic studies have also been undertaken focusing on variations in ATP binding cassette (ABC) transporter genes, based on the assumption that diminished functions of hepatocellular efflux transporters and subsequent drug clearance might critically influence the level of exposure to drug compounds. Genetic variations in *ABCB1*, which encodes P-glycoprotein 1 (also referred to as MDR1) have been associated with decreased risk of DILI induced by nevirapine in various independent cohorts.[23–25] The rs1045642 polymorphism found to have a protective effect on nevirapine hepatotoxicity was not confirmed to have a similar effect on atorvastatin hepatotoxicity in Japanese patients. Instead a different *ABCB1* polymorphism (rs2032582) was reported as a genetic risk factor for atorvastatin.[26] Results relating to the effect of genetic variations in the *ABCC2* gene, which encodes the MDR2 transporter, are still controversial.[4,27,28] However, *ABCC2* is still of interest after the detection of several SNPs in the region of this gene in a large GWA study. These SNPs were the most associated SNPs located in the drug-metabolizing genes covered in the study, although none reached genome-wide significance.[29]

GENOME-WIDE ASSOCIATION STUDIES

Introduction of the SNP array technology has shifted the focus of DILI genetic studies from conventional CG studies to GWA studies over the last decade. The GWA study concept brought great anticipation because of its potential to widen the understanding of DILI through the identification of genetic variations located in genes currently unknown to play a mechanistic role in hepatotoxicity. Surprisingly, although, genetic variations in drug-metabolizing genes identified in earlier CG studies have not been confirmed in any GWA study. In fact, DILI associations with genome-wide significance identified through GWA studies to date are almost exclusively genetic variations in the HLA region on chromosome 6 or tagSNPs in strong linkage disequilibrium with specific HLA alleles.

HLA Risk Alleles

More than a dozen different drugs associated with DILI have been linked to increased risk in carriers of specific HLA alleles, including both HLA class I and II alleles (**Table 2**).[30–39] Intriguingly, causative agents without any apparent connection in terms of chemical structure or pharmacologic targets share HLA risk alleles. For example, the presence of HLA-DRB1*15:01-DQB1*06:02 increases the risk of DILI induced by amoxicillin-clavulanate and lumiracoxib, whereas HLA-DRB1*07:01 carriers are at higher risk of developing DILI caused by ximelagatran and lapatinib.[30,35–38] In contrast, the presence of HLA-DRB1*07 has been associated with protection against

Table 2
Genetic polymorphisms associated with idiosyncratic drug-induced liver injury identified in genome-wide association studies

Locus	Causative Drug	Odds Ratio	Reference
HLA			
A*02:01	Amoxicillin-clavulanate	2.3	Lucena et al,[30] 2011
A*33:01	Various drugs	2.6	Nicoletti et al,[31] 2017
A*33:01	Terbinafine	40.5	Nicoletti et al,[31] 2017
A*33:01	Fenofibrate	58.7	Nicoletti et al,[31] 2017
A*33:01	Ticlopidine	163.1	Nicoletti et al,[31] 2017
B*35:02	Minocycline	29.6	Urban et al,[32] 2017
B*57:01	Flucloxacillin	81/37	Daly et al,[33] 2009; Nicoletti et al,[34] 2019
DRB1*07	Ximelagatran	4.4	Kindmark et al,[35] 2008
DRB1*07:01	Lapatinib	NA	Spraggs et al,[36] 2011; Parham et al,[37] 2016
DRB1*15:01	Lumiracoxib	5.0	Singer et al,[38] 2008
DRB1*15:01-DQB1*06:02	Amoxicillin-clavulanate	2.8	Lucena et al,[30] 2011
DRB1*16:01-DQB1*05:02	Flupirtine	18.7	Nicoletti et al,[39] 2016
Non-HLA			
rs72631567	Various	2.0	Nicoletti et al,[31] 2017
rs116561224	Statins	5.4	Nicoletti et al,[31] 2017
ST6GAL1, rs10937275	Flucloxacillin	4.1	Daly et al,[33] 2009
PTPN22, rs2476601	Various	1.4–1.9	Cirulli et al,[46] 2019
FAM65B, rs10946737	Rifampicin	3.4	Petros et al,[49] 2016
ERN1, rs199650082	Efavirenz	18.2	Petros et al,[50] 2017
lincRNA, rs4842407	Efavirenz + anti-TBC	5.4	Petros et al,[50] 2017

Abbreviations: NA, not available; TBC, tuberculosis.

DILI caused by amoxicillin-clavulanate, although this finding has not been confirmed through GWA studies.[40] The fact that the same HLA allele is associated with increased DILI risk for one drug, while providing protection against DILI due to another drug, is in line with the hapten theory, and differences in the DNA sequence translated into amino acid variation in the HLA binding groove will restrict the type of neoantigens (produced by the drug-protein complex) that can bind. Flucloxacillin hepatotoxicity has been associated with the HLA class I allele B*57:01 and recently also with B*57:03, a relatively rare allele in white patients.[33,34] These alleles have not been confirmed as risk factors for other forms of DILI up to now, although HLA-B*57:01 carriage has been associated with increased risk of transaminase elevations in clinical trials of pazopanib treatment in patients with cancer.[41] Nevertheless, HLA-B*57:01 is strongly associated with risk of abacavir hypersensitivity, but the mechanistic role of abacavir differs somewhat from that of flucloxacillin.[42] Abacavir has been demonstrated to bind directly and specifically to the HLA-B*57:01 protein and cause an inappropriate immune response, whereas flucloxacillin seems to bind covalently to endogenous proteins resulting in the presentation of modified self-peptides to T cells.[43,44]

In search for common DILI risk factors independent of the causative agent, a large GWA study comparing DILI patients of European ancestry with an array of causative agents and population-matched controls was performed, but no such common genetic risk factors, including in the HLA region, were found.[29] It is possible that the lack of results stemmed from the large proportion of patients with amoxicillin-clavlanate and flucloxacillin hepatotoxicity, because a similar GWA study a few years later including 862 DILI patients with hepatotoxicity ownig to various causative agents (excluding amoxicillin-clavulanate and flucloxacillin) was more successful in terms of identification of risk alleles. This study was the first to identify a common genetic variation rs114577328 (a proxy for HLA-A*33:01) as a risk factor for various drugs, including terbinafine, fenofibrate, and ticlopidine.[31] Interestingly, ticlopidine-induced hepatotoxicity, particularly with cholestatic presentation, in Japanese patients has previously been associated with HLA-A*33:03 in a CG study.[45] The HLA-A*33:03 allele is very similar to HLA-A*33:01, and the corresponding proteins differ in only two amino acid positions. However, HLA-A*33:03 is rare in Europeans but is relatively common in Japanese.

Non-HLA Genes

The rs2476601 SNP located on chromosome 1 in lymphoid-specific protein tyrosine phosphatase non-receptor type 22 (PTPN22) is an identified non-HLA association with genome-wide significance. The association identified in a large cohort of 2048 DILI patients was robust and remained across a broad range of implicated drugs and different ethnic backgrounds. Hence, it can be seen as the first identified general risk association for DILI. The effect size of rs2476601 was, however, relatively modest, although it increased with joint carriage of known HLA risk alleles, such as DRB1*15:01 and A*02:01 for amoxicillin-clavulanate.[46] In fact, rs2476601 was detected in an earlier GWA study of amoxicillin-clavlanate DILI as potentially involved in this form of DILI, although not reaching genome-wide significance.[30] The finding of rs2476601 is particularly interesting because this polymorphism predisposes carriers to several autoimmune diseases, as well as being associated with alterations in the composition of intestinal microbiota in inflammatory bowel disease.[47,48] PTPN22 is involved in both T and B cell signaling and subsequent regulatory functions, and it has been hypothesized that the rs2476601 variant may be involved in reducing immune tolerance in DILI patients.[46,47] Tendencies toward enrichment in DILI patients for other genetic non-HLA variants have also been detected (see **Table 2**), although few have been validated in independent studies.[31,33,49,50]

GENETIC TESTING FOR DRUG-INDUCED LIVER INJURY IN CLINICAL PRACTICE

The identification of genetic predisposition to DILI is of paramount importance to widen the understanding of the underlying mechanism of DILI. But, is this information of any use for DILI management in clinical practice? The usefulness for pre-prescription genotyping to identify susceptible individuals and consequently reduce the number of DILI cases is limited, because the low incidence rate of DILI inevitably leads to a low positive predictive value (PPV) for identified genetic variations. One of the largest effect sizes for HLA risk alleles in DILI is that of HLA-B*57:01 for flucloxacillin, with B*57:01 carriers found to be associated with an 80-fold increased risk of developing DILI if treated with flucloxacillin.[33] Based on reported incidence data from epidemiologic studies, it has been estimated that 13,500 subjects would need to be screened to prevent one flucloxacillin-induced liver injury case.[51] Unlike flucloxacillin with a PPV of 0.12% for HLA-B*57:01, abacavir has a PPV of 48% for hypersensitivity reactions in the presence of the same HLA allele, which makes pre-prescription genetic testing a very useful tool that is now mandatory for abacavir in many countries.[52]

Moreover, many identified HLA risk alleles for DILI have a high negative predictive value (>95%), which enables the use of HLA information in DILI diagnosis.[53] That is, in patients suspected of DILI caused by a drug with an identified HLA risk allele, information on the patient's HLA genotype can support or refute the diagnosis of DILI. Similarly, in situations where DILI is suspected and the patient has been exposed to multiple drugs with hepatotoxicity potential before the hepatic reaction, HLA genotyping can aid clinical decision-making by indicating which drug is the most likely causative agent, provided that HLA risk alleles are available for the drugs in question. Such a decision is important to make and to communicate to the patient to avoid future inadvertent reexposure to the causative agent, which could lead to a new and at times more severe DILI episode for the patient.

An accurate DILI diagnosis obtained at an early stage of the disease progression is crucial, because withdrawing the causative agent is one of the most important interventions to decrease the risk of a severe outcome. Furthermore, wrongly diagnosed DILI or incorrect identification of the causative agent may lead to unnecessary drug withdrawal of an effective medication, which can have important implications for the patient. Symptoms of DILI and autoimmune hepatitis (AIH) often overlap and there are no pathognomonic features for either of these conditions. Distinguishing DILI with concomitant autoimmune features from preexisting or new-onset AIH can therefore be diagnostically challenging.[54] Similar to DILI, genetic predisposition to AIH has been identified in the form of specific HLA alleles. Several CG studies have found associations between AIH type 1 and primarily HLA-DRB1*03:01, but also DRB1*04:01 in Europeans.[55,56] These associations have since been confirmed in a GWA study.[57] It should be noted that limited genetic studies have been performed on idiopathic AIH populations outside of Europe and North America. Hence, the aforementioned AIH risk alleles require further studies to determine their applicability to patients of non-European descent. Nevertheless, HLA genotypes have been suggested to be strong enough to be considered as diagnostic criteria for idiopathic AIH in the revised diagnostic scoring system designed by the International AIH Group.[58]

In contrast, DILI patients presenting autoimmune features, such as positive autoantibody titers, do not seem to be enriched in DRB1*03:01 or 04:01 carriage.[56,59] These differences could be diagnostically useful. When the physician is faced with a liver injury case in which a temporal relationship between drug intake and start of liver-related symptoms exists, and the patient presents with positive autoantibodies, such as antinuclear antibody (ANA), anti-smooth muscle antibody, anti-liver-kidney microsomal antibody (anti-LKM), or raised immunoglobulin G (IgG), HLA genotyping could help distinguishing DILI with concomitant autoimmune features from preexisting or new-onset AIH. In addition to current diagnostic procedures, the presence of AIH HLA risk alleles (such as DRB1*03:01 or 04:01) would support the diagnosis of AIH, whereas the presence of specific DILI HLA risk alleles (such as B*35:02 for minocycline) would support that of DILI with autoimmune features (**Fig. 1**).

The frequency of currently identified HLA risk alleles in DILI, such as DRB1*15:01 for amoxicillin-clavulanate, B*57:01 for flucloxacillin, and B*35:02 for minocycline in DILI patients and the general population are similar to the corresponding frequencies for the presence of ANA autoantibodies, raised immunoglobulin G levels, and anti-LKM autoantibodies, respectively.[60] Hence, HLA genotyping in the examples above would have similar performance characteristics to those of ANA, IgG, and anti-LKM testing, which are well-established diagnostic criteria for idiopathic AIH.[61] The incorporation of HLA genotyping in this clinical setting can enhance both accuracy and

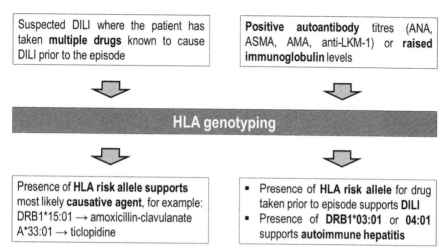

Fig. 1. Use of HLA genotyping in idiosyncratic drug-induced liver injury in clinical practice. The applicability of the HLA alleles included in the figure is currently limited to white European ancestry.

confidence of the diagnosis. This is important in terms of appropriate treatment care for the patient, because AIH mostly requires long-term immunosuppressive treatment, whereas DILI with autoimmune features often can be self-limiting after drug withdrawal.[60]

SUMMARY AND FUTURE PERSPECTIVES

The search for genetic predisposition to DILI has resulted in various identified polymorphisms in drug-metabolizing genes through CG studies, of which few have been confirmed in more recent GWA studies. This may to some degree depend on the fact that CG studies tend to have a higher statistical power than GWA studies, with the latter having a very high threshold for genome-wide significance owing to the large number of simultaneously screened SNPs. Nevertheless, there is evidence to support the idea that the immune system is a vital component in DILI development because of the identification of specific HLA alleles enriched in DILI patients. However, these HLA risk alleles are associated with low PPVs and therefore do not meet the threshold for clinical application in the form of pre-prescription genetic screening to prevent DILI. Nevertheless, incorporated into the diagnostic process information on the presence or absence of HLA risk alleles can support or refute a DILI diagnosis, provide guidance on the most likely causative agent in patients exposed to multiple drugs before the development of liver damage, and assist in distinguishing DILI with autoimmune features from idiopathic AIH. Hence, HLA genotyping can enhance both accuracy and confidence in the DILI diagnostic process.

Despite considerable progress in the area of genetic predisposition to DILI over the last decades, the final goal is not yet reached and the search will continue. Whole-genome sequencing offers an alternative to GWA studies that enables the circumvention of inherent methodological limitations to the latter, such as detection of rare genetic variations that could have considerably larger effects on DILI. But technological advances alone are not likely to find the genetic answers in DILI. Because of the low incidence rate of DILI, collaborations are essential to overcome the hurdle of small cohort sizes faced by individual hospital units.

Recent collaborations between European and North American groups have demonstrated the power of joint efforts and set a good example for future DILI studies.

ACKNOWLEDGMENTS

We acknowledge the support from the European Cooperation in Science & Technology (COST) Action CA17112 Prospective European Drug-Induced Liver Injury Network. C.S and R.J.A. are members of COST Action CA17112.

REFERENCES

1. Ingelman-Sundberg M, Sim SC, Gomez A, et al. Influence of cytochrome P450 polymorphisms on drug therapies: pharmacogenetic, pharmacoepigenetic and clinical aspects. Pharmacol Ther 2007;116:496–526.
2. Yu K, Geng X, Chen M, et al. High daily dose and being a substrate of cytochrome P450 enzymes are two important predictors of drug-induced liver injury. Drug Metab Dispos 2014;42:744–50.
3. Aithal GP, Day CP, Leathart JB, et al. Relationship of polymorphism in CYP2C9 to genetic susceptibility to diclofenac-induced hepatitis. Pharmacogenetics 2000; 10:511–8.
4. Daly AK, Aithal GP, Leathart JB, et al. Genetic susceptibility to diclofenac-induced hepatotoxicity: contribution of UGT2B7, CYP2C, and ABCC2 genotypes. Gastroenterology 2007;132:272–81.
5. Pachkoria K, Lucena MI, Ruiz-Cabello F, et al. Genetic polymorphisms of CYP2C9 and CYP2C19 are not related to drug-induced idiosyncratic liver injury (DILI). Br J Pharmacol 2007;150:808–15.
6. Ariyoshi N, Iga Y, Hirata K, et al. Enhanced susceptibility of HLA-mediated ticlopidine-induced idiosyncratic hepatotoxicity by CYP2B6 polymorphism in Japanese. Drug Metab Pharmacokinet 2010;25:298–306.
7. Yimer G, Amogne W, Habtewold A, et al. High plasma efavirenz level and CYP2B6*6 are associated with efavirenz-based HAART-induced liver injury in the treatment of naïve HIV patients from Ethiopia: a prospective cohort stuy. Pharmacogenomics J 2012;12:499–506.
8. Zhao M, Zhang T, Li G, et al. Associations of CYP2C9 and CYP2A6 polymorphisms with the concentration of valproate and its hepatotoxin metabolites and valproate-induced hepatotoxicity. Basic Clin Pharmacol Toxicol 2017;121: 138–43.
9. Huang YS, Chern HD, Su WJ, et al. Cytochrome P450 2E1 genotype and the susceptibility to antituberculosis drug-induced hepatitis. Hepatology 2003;37: 924–30.
10. Wang FJ, Wang Y, Niu T, et al. Update meta-analysis of the CYP2E1 RsaI/PstI and DraI polymorphisms and risk of antituberculosis drug-induced hepatotoxicity: evidence from 26 studies. J Clin Pharm Ther 2016;41:334–40.
11. Lazarska KE, Dekker SJ, Vermeulen NPE, et al. Effect of UGT2B7*2 and CYP2CB*4 polymorphisms on diclofenac metabolism. Toxicol Lett 2018; 284:70–8.
12. Acuña G, Foernzler D, Leong D, et al. Pharmacogenetic analysis of adverse drug effect reveals genetic variant for susceptibility to liver toxicity. Pharmacogenomics J 2002;2:327–34.

13. Du H, Chen X, Fang Y, et al. Slow N-acetyltransferase 2 genotype contributes to anti-tuberculosis drug-induced hepatotoxicity: a meta-analysis. Mol Biol Rep 2013;40:3591–6.
14. Zhang M, Wang S, Wilffert B, et al. The association between the NAT2 genetic polymorphisms and risk of DILI during anti-TB treatment: a systematic review and meta-analysis. Br J Clin Pharmacol 2018;84:2747–60.
15. Nicoletti P, Devarbhavi H, Goel A, et al. Genome-wide association study (GWAS) to identify genetic risk factors that increase susceptibility to anti-tuberculosis drug-induced liver injury (ATDILI). Hepatology 2017;66(Suppl 1):25A.
16. Simon T, Becquemont L, Mary-Krause M, et al. Combined glutathione-S-transferase M1 and T1 genetic polymorphism and tacrine hepatotoxicity. Clin Pharmacol Ther 2000;67:432–7.
17. Watanabe I, Tomita A, Shimizu M, et al. A study to survey susceptible genetic factors responsible for troglitazone-associated hepatotoxicity in Japanese patients with type 2 diabetes mellitus. Clin Pharmacol Ther 2003;73:435–55.
18. Gupta VH, Singh M, Amarapurkar DN, et al. Association of GST null genotypes with anti-tuberculosis drug induced hepatotoxicity in Western Indian population. Ann Hepatol 2013;12:959–65.
19. Lucena MI, Andrade RJ, Martínez C, et al. Glutathione S-transferase m1 and t1 null genotypes increase susceptibility to idiosyncratic drug-induced liver injury. Hepatology 2008;48:588–96.
20. Xiang Y, Ma L, Wu W, et al. The incidence of liver injury in Uyghur patients treated for TB in Xinjiang Uyghur autonomous region, China, and its association with hepatic enzyme polymorphisms nat2, cyp2e1, gstm1 and gstt1. PLoS One 2014;9: e85905.
21. Monteiro TP, El-Jaick KB, Jeovanio-Silva AL, et al. The roles of GSTM1 and GSTT1 null genotypes and other predictors in anti-tuberculosis drug-induced liver injury. J Clin Pharm Ther 2012;37:712–8.
22. Bhattacharjee P, Paul S, Banerjee M, et al. Functional compensation of glutathione S-transferase M1 (GSTM1) null by another GST superfamily member, GSTM2. Sci Rep 2013;3:2704.
23. Haas DW, Bartlett JA, Andersen JW, et al. Pharmacogenetics of nevirapine-associated hepatotoxicity: an adult AIDS clinical trials group collaboration. Clin Infect Dis 2006;43:783–6.
24. Ritchie MD, Haas DW, Motsinger AA, et al. Drug transporter and metabolizing enzyme gene variants and nonnucleoside reverse-transcriptase inhibitor hepatotoxicity. Clin Infect Dis 2006;15:779–82.
25. Ciccacci C, Borgiani P, Ceffa S, et al. Nevirapine-induced hepatotoxicity and pharmacogenetics: a retrospective study in a population from Mozambique. Pharmacogenomics 2010;11:23–31.
26. Fukunaga K, Nakagawa H, Ishikawa T, et al. ABCB1 polymorphism is associated with atorvastatin-induced liver injury in Japanese population. BMC Genet 2016; 17:79.
27. Choi JH, Ahn BM, Yi J, et al. MRP2 haplotypes confer differential susceptibility to toxic liver injury. Pharmacogenet Genomics 2007;17:403–15.
28. Ulzurrun E, Stephens C, Ruiz-Cabello F, et al. Selected ABCB1, ABCB4 and ABCC2 polymorphisms do not enhance the risk of drug-induced hepatotoxicity in a Spanish cohort. PLoS One 2014;9:e94675.
29. Urban TJ, Shen Y, Stolz A, et al. Limited contribution of common genetic variants to risk for liver injury due to a variety of drugs. Pharmacogenet Genomics 2012; 22:784–95.

30. Lucena M, Molokhia M, Shen Y, et al. Susceptibility to amoxicillin-clavulanate-induced liver injury is influenced by multiple HLA class I and class II alleles. Gastroenterology 2011;141:338–47.

31. Nicoletti P, Aithal GP, Björnsson ES, et al. Association of liver injury from specific drugs, or groups of drugs, with polymorphisms in HLA and other genes in a genome-wide association study. Gastroenterology 2017;152:1078–89.

32. Urban TJ, Nicoletti P, Chalasani N, et al. Minocycline hepatotoxicity: clinical characterization and identification of HLA-B*35:02 as a risk factor. J Hepatol 2017;67: 137–44.

33. Daly AK, Donaldson PT, Bhatnagar P, et al. HLA-B*5701 genotype is a major determinant of drug-induced liver injury due to flucloxacillin. Nat Genet 2009; 41:816–9.

34. Nicoletti P, Aithal GP, Chamberlain TC, et al. Drug-induced liver injury due to flucloxacillin: relevance of multiple human leukocyte antigen alleles. Clin Pharmacol Ther 2019;106(1):245–53.

35. Kindmark A, Jawaid A, Harbron CG, et al. Genome-wide pharmacogenetic investigation of a hepatic adverse event without clinical signs of immunopathology suggests an underlying immune pathogenesis. Pharmacogenomics J 2008;8: 186–95.

36. Spraggs CF, Budde LR, Briley LP, et al. HLA-DQA1*02:01 is a major risk factor for lapatinib-induced hepatotoxicity in women with advanced breast cancer. J Clin Oncol 2011;29:667–73.

37. Parham LR, Briley LP, Li L, et al. Comprehensive genome-wide evaluation of lapatinib-induced liver injury yields a single genetic signal centered on known risk allele HLA-DRB1*07:01. Pharmacogenomics J 2016;16:180–5.

38. Singer JB, Lewitzky S, Leroy E, et al. A genome-wide study identifies HLA alleles associated with lumiracoxib-related liver injury. Nat Genet 2008;42:711–4.

39. Nicoletti P, Werk AN, Sawle A, et al. HLA-DRB1*16:01-DQB1*05:02 is a novel genetic risk factor for flupirtine-induced liver injury. Pharmacogenet Genomics 2016;26:218–24.

40. Donaldson PT, Daly AK, Henderson J, et al. Human leucocyte antigen class II genotype is susceptibility and resistance to co-amoxiclav-induced liver injury. J Hepatol 2010;53:1049–53.

41. Xu CF, Johnson T, Wang X, et al. HLA-B*57:01 confers susceptibility to pazopanib-associated liver injury in patients with cancer. Clin Cancer Res 2016;22:1371–7.

42. Mallal S, Nolan D, Witt C, et al. Association between presence of HLA-B*5701, HLA-DR7, and HLA-DQ3 and hypersensitivity to HIV-1 reverse-transcriptase inhibitor abacavir. Lancet 2002;359:727–32.

43. Illing PT, Vivian JP, Dudek NL, et al. Immune self-reactivity triggered by drug-modified HLA-peptide repertoire. Nature 2012;486:554–8.

44. Monshi MM, Faulkner L, Gibson A, et al. Human leukocyte antigen (HLA)-B*57:01-restricted activation of drug-specific T cells provides the immunological basis for flucloxacillin-induced liver injury. Hepatology 2013;57:727–39.

45. Hirata K, Takagi H, Yamamoto M, et al. Ticlopidine-induced hepatotoxicity is associated with specific human leukocyte antigen genomic subtypes in Japanese patients: a preliminary case-control study. Pharmacogenomics J 2008;8: 29–33.

46. Cirulli ET, Nicoletti P, Abramson K, et al. A missense variant in PTPN22 is a risk factor for drug-induced liver injury. Gastroenterology 2019;156(6):1707–16.e2.

47. Vang T, Nielsen J, Burn GL. A switch-variant model integrates the functions of an autoimmune variant of the phosphatase PTPN22. Sci Signal 2018;11:eaat0936.
48. Yilmaz B, Spalinger MR, Biedermann L, et al. The presence of genetic risk variants within PTPN2 and PTPN22 is associated with intestinal microbiota alteration in Swiss IBD cohort patients. PLoS One 2018;13:e0199664.
49. Petros Z, Lee MT, Takahashi A, et al. Genome-wide association and replication study of anti-tuberculosis drugs-induced liver toxicity. BMC Genomics 2016; 17:755.
50. Petros Z, Lee MT, Takahashi A, et al. Genome-wide association and replication study of hepatotoxicity induced by antiretrovirals alone or with concomitant anti-tuberculosis drugs. OMICS 2017;21:207–16.
51. Alfirevic A, Pirmohamed M. Predictive genetic testing for drug-induced liver injury: considerations of clinical utility. Clin Pharamcol Ther 2012;92:376–80.
52. Mallal S, Phillips E, Carosi G, et al. HLA-B*57:01 screening for hypersensitivity to abacavir. N Engl J Med 2008;358:568–79.
53. Aithal GP. Pharmacogenetic testing in idiosyncratic drug-induced liver injury: current role in clinical practice. Liver Int 2015;35:1801–8.
54. Castiella A, Zapata E, Lucena MI, et al. Drug-induced autoimmune liver disease: a diagnostic dilemma of an increasingly reported disease. World J Hepatol 2014; 6:160–8.
55. Strettell MD, Donaldson PT, Thomson LJ, et al. Allelic basis for HLA-encoded susceptibility to type 1 autoimmune hepatitis. Gastroenterology 1997;112:2028–35.
56. Stephens C, Castiella A, Gomez-Moreno EM, et al. Autoantibody presentation in drug-induced liver injury and idiopathic autoinmune hepatitis: the influence of human leucocyte antigen alleles. Pharmacogenet Genomics 2016;26:414–22.
57. de Boer YS, van Gerven NM, Zwiers A, et al. Genome-wide association study identifies variants associated with autoimmune hepatitis type 1. Gastroenterology 2014;147:443–52.
58. Alvarez F, Berg PA, Bianchi FB, et al. International autoimmune hepatitis group report: review of criteria for diagnosis of autoimmune hepatitis. J Hepatol 1999; 31:929–38.
59. de Boer YS, Kosinski AS, Urban TJ, et al. Features of autoimmune hepatitis in patients with drug-induced liver injury. Clin Gastroenterol Hepatol 2017;15:103–12.
60. Kaliyaperumal K, Grove JI, Delahay RM, et al. Pharmacogenomics of drug-induced liver injury (DILI): molecular biology to clinical applications. J Hepatol 2018;69:948–57.
61. Hennes EM, Zeniya M, Czaja AJ, et al. Simplified criteria for the diagnosis of autoinmune hepatitis. Hepatology 2008;48:169–76.

Drug Hepatotoxicity
Causality Assessment

Allyce Caines, MD*, Dilip Moonka, MD*

KEYWORDS

- Causality • RUCAM • Naranjo • Mario and Victorino • Expert opinion

KEY POINTS

- Causality assessment for the cause of drug-induced liver injury (DILI) can be done using a standardized method such as Roussel Uclaf Causality Assessment Method, a clinician's clinical judgment, or by expert opinion when available.
- Prompt recognition of the culprit drug or toxin decreases the risk of progression to chronic liver injury or acute liver failure.
- There is room for improvement in causality assessment with the identification of liver- and drug/toxin-specific biomarkers and further understanding of clinical and genetic risk factors and the contribution of underlying liver disease.

INTRODUCTION

Drug-induced liver injury (DILI) remains a leading global health problem and is the number one cause of acute liver failure in the United States. DILI can be dose dependent as seen in acetaminophen overdose or idiosyncratic where the injury can be specific to a particular individual. Patients are often prescribed several medications and may also be using over-the-counter medications or herbal supplements. Almost any medication or herbal supplement has the potential to cause liver injury. The challenge lies in distinguishing a specific drug or toxin as the cause of injury. Prompt recognition of a culprit drug as the cause of liver injury is the most important aspect in hepatotoxicity management, as it decreases the risk of progression to acute liver failure or chronic liver injury.[1]

DILI is a diagnosis that relies on the knowledge of patterns of injury associated with specific medications and herbal supplements. During the process of determining causality, other common causes of liver disease must be excluded. There is no specific diagnostic test that can establish causality for DILI.[2] Several assessment tools have been developed in an attempt to aide physicians in the diagnosis of drug hepatotoxicity and the assignment of causality to a specific medication or toxin. This article

---

Henry Ford Hospital, 2799 West Grand Boulevard, Suite K7, Detroit, MI 48202, USA
* Corresponding authors.
E-mail addresses: acaines1@hfhs.org (A.C.); DMOONKA1@hfhs.org (D.M.)

Clin Liver Dis 24 (2020) 25–35
https://doi.org/10.1016/j.cld.2019.09.001
1089-3261/20/© 2019 Elsevier Inc. All rights reserved.

liver.theclinics.com

reviews the most commonly used causality assessment methods including their strengths and limitations.

CAUSALITY ASSESSMENT

Causality assessment entails the evaluation of the likelihood that a particular drug or toxin is the cause of liver injury.[3] Diagnosis of DILI requires a high level of suspicion. Polypharmacy and comorbid conditions can complicate DILI diagnosis.[4] Methods to determine causality often rely on careful delineation between the onset of the adverse event in relation to starting the medication (challenge) and the timing of resolution in relation to stopping the medication (dechallenge).[2] Causality is further strengthened if there is recurrent DILI on reexposure (rechallenge).[2] A clinician may also find knowledge of hypersensitivity signs/symptoms, known drug allergies, and previous information on the occurrence of a similar adverse event helpful in assessing causality.

As there are no reliable biomarkers for the causality assessment of DILI, several standardized systems have been proposed to assess the relationship between drugs and the appearance of DILI. Attempts have been made to standardize causality assessment methods in DILI. The systems that are currently available to aide in determining causality include algorithms or scales, probabilistic methods, and expert judgment.[4] This article will focus on algorithms, scales, and expert judgement.

ROUSSEL UCLAF CAUSALITY ASSESSMENT METHOD

The Roussel Uclaf Causality Assessment Method (RUCAM) was introduced in 1993 and was the first causality assessment method specific to liver injury. The strength of RUCAM is that it was the first CAM to include the pattern of liver injury as a criterion for causality assessment. The R ratio is the first value to be calculated in the RUCAM assessment and is used to define the hepatic injury as hepatocellular, cholestatic, or mixed. Recognizing the latter may occur after a longer withdrawal period and resolves more slowly.[4] The R ratio is calculated at the beginning of the liver injury by dividing the alanine aminotransferase by the alkaline phosphatase, using multiples of the upper limit of the normal range for both values. Once the R ratio has been determined and the pattern of injury defined, a RUCAM score can be calculated.[5] Within RUCAM, points are awarded for 7 components where the criteria for scoring the first 3 of the 7 components are determined by the R ratio. The 7 components include the following: time to onset of the injury following the start of the drug, subsequent course of the injury after stopping the drug, specific risk factors (age, alcohol use, pregnancy), use of other medications with a potential for liver injury, exclusion of other causes of liver disease, known potential for hepatotoxicity of the implicated drug, and response to rechallenge. These criteria were developed from a series of DILI cases, with positive rechallenge recognized as the gold standard to confirm the diagnosis.[6] The overall score is then used to categorize the likelihood that the liver injury is due to a specific medication as: excluded, unlikely, possible, probable, and highly probable.[2]

RUCAM has been tested repeatedly for accuracy, reproducibility, and interobserver variability and has shown high sensitivity, specificity, positive predictive value (PPV), and negative predictive value (NPV). Based on 77 case reports with positive rechallenge, RUCAM was found to have a sensitivity (86%), specificity (89%), PPV (93%), and NPV (78%).[7] In regard to reproducibility, in a study by Danan G and colleagues, 4 external assessors independently evaluated 50 DILI cases with RUCAM with very low interobserver variability with no disagreement in 84% of cases that they assessed.[8] The strength of RUCAM is that cases can be assessed prospectively as soon as DILI is suspected or retrospectively when additional data is available. RUCAM can identify DILI cases early in clinical drug development enabling companies and regulatory agencies to propose measures to minimize the risk of severe hepatic reactions.[9] In cases where different drugs or toxins are taken concomitantly, RUCAM allows identification of the most likely offending product.[9,10]

LIMITATIONS OF ROUSSEL UCLAF CAUSALITY ASSESSMENT METHOD

Critics of RUCAM note several limitations in its use. RUCAM is not commonly used in clinical practice as many of the factors included are not well described and are open to variable interpretation.[4] The first step in using RUCAM is calculation of the R value. The R value is used to define DILI as hepatocellular, cholestatic, or mixed. It is important to note that the R value is calculated using one set of enzyme values, and the type of injury may change along the course of the illness. The calculation can vary between users, as some may use enzyme values from the first analytical test, whereas others may use peak values.[4]

RUCAM efficiency depends on the amount of available data for the case as well as where along the clinical course of DILI a clinician is evaluating a patient. Early suspicion of DILI can lead to a low RUCAM probability score due to lack of data such as response to dechallenge. In cases of acute liver failure (ALF) leading rapidly to death or liver transplantation, the course of alanine aminotransferase elevations may not be available or may be unreliable. In this and many other ways, assessing causality in ALF is very difficult.[5] In cases with an aberrant reaction course, such as long-term cholestasis or cases of ALF leading rapidly to death or liver transplantation, the RUCAM scale tends to give lower probability scores leading to the underdiagnosis of cases in this category.[11]

RUCAM also incorporates rechallenge as part of its scoring system. Inadvertent reexposure occasionally occurs when a patient restarts a medication without understanding its potential harm or a physician prescribes a medication unaware of a previous adverse episode. Rechallenge is rarely deliberately done however due to potential risks. RUCAM does not include liver biopsy findings or immunoallergic features that could potentially aide in the clinician's assessment of causality. Presence of biopsy findings that suggests DILI such as demarcated perivenular (acinar zone 3) necrosis, minimal hepatitis with canalicular cholestasis, poorly developed portal inflammatory reaction, abundant neutrophils, abundant eosinophils, epithelioid-cell granulomas, microvesicular steatosis, and the presence of drug deposits (vitamin A autofluorescence) could possibly upgrade the causality assessment score.[12,13] The use of older age as a risk factor in RUCAM has been disputed. In RUCAM, age greater than 55 years is considered a risk factor. However, data from a large cohort indicated that older age does not predispose to overall DILI but can be a predictor of cholestatic damage, whereas younger age seems to be related to hepatocellular pattern or injury.[14] The 7 domains of the RUCAM scale are also weighted differently toward the final calculated score. The weighting of the domains is based on expert opinion and has not been derived from statistical approaches. This could potentially lead to biased or incorrect causality results.

MARIA AND VICTORINO SCALE

The Maria and Victorino scale (M&V) was developed by investigators from Portugal in an effort to develop a simplified scoring system to overcome the complexity of RUCAM. The scale includes 5 components: time to onset of injury following start of the drug, exclusion of other causes of liver disease, extrahepatic manifestations (rash, fever, eosinophilia, cytopenias), known potential for hepatotoxicity of the implicated drug, and response to rechallenge. The scale incorporates clinical elements of extrahepatic manifestations of DILI.[15] The relative weights of the 5 elements in the assessment of causality were altered from their weighting in RUCAM. However, as RUCAM, the weighting of each element is subjective. The overall score corresponds to 5 probability degrees: definite, probable, possible, unlikely, and excluded. Key differences from RUCAM include the exclusion of points for risk factors such as age, alcohol use, and pregnancy and the subtraction of points for other medications (whether they are hepatotoxins or not). The M&V scale was validated using real and fictitious cases and compared with the classification of 3 external experts. The comparison showed 84% agreement between the M&V scale and expert opinions.[16]

LIMITATIONS OF MARIA AND VICTORINO SCALE

Several limitations have made the M&V scale a less favorable scale to use in causality assessment. The scale classifies cases as definite only when positive rechallenge and hypersensitivity features are present. The scale does not clearly define what constitutes fever or relevant rash. The difficulty and impracticality of rechallenge has been discussed earlier. Both rechallenge and repeat DILI occur infrequently in a patient with an initial case of DILI. The scale has also been shown to perform poorly in atypical cases, such as those with unusually long latency periods or those leading to chronic evolution after drug withdrawal.[4]

The M&V scale also includes prior knowledge of the hepatotoxic potential of a potential offending drug. The score in this category will be limited by the clinician's knowledge of whether there is at least one case report of injury due to the medication. Also, drugs with more than 5 years on the market and no documented hepatotoxicity potential are given a lower score. Unlike RUCAM, the M&V scale does not differentiate between hepatocellular, cholestatic, or mixed injury. There is a potential for false-negative judgments in cholestatic DILI cases because the pattern of liver injury is not taken into consideration in the M&V scale.[17]

NARANJO ADVERSE DRUG REACTIONS PROBABILITY SCALE

The Naranjo adverse drug reactions probability scale (NADRPS) was developed in 1991 to help standardize assessment of causality for all adverse drug reactions. This scale was designed for use in controlled trials and registration studies of new medications and not specifically designed for DILI.[18] The NADRPS involves 10 "yes", "no", or "unknown/inapplicable" questions. Based on the total score, a probability of definite, probable, or doubtful is given.[19] The NADRPS questions that are relevant to idiosyncratic reactions include the following: Did the adverse event appear after the drug was given? Did the adverse reaction improve when the drug was discontinued? Has the patient had a similar reaction to the drug or related agent in the past? Are there previous conclusive reports of this reaction? Rechallenge is also addressed in this scale with the following question: Did the adverse reaction reappear on readministration of the drug? Several questions in NADRPS are not applicable to DILI or are difficult to answer in a clinical setting. An example of such a question is the following: Was the drug detected in the blood or other fluids in toxic concentrations? It is known that testing of drug levels is rarely helpful in idiosyncratic DILI. The question of whether the reaction worsened on increasing the dose is often difficult to answer with the information available at that time of DILI evaluation. NADRPS also includes the following question: Did the adverse reaction reappear on administration of placebo, which is typically not applicable to the setting in which a clinician is evaluating a patient with

DILI. Advantages of NADRPS include simplicity, wide applicability, and easier use compared with RUCAM.

LIMITATIONS OF NARANJO ADVERSE DRUG REACTIONS PROBABILITY SCALE

There are limitations in the use of NADRPS scale in addition to the fact that the scale is not specific to DILI. The questions in the NADRPS scale are not weighted for the most relevant elements in determining the likelihood of DILI such as time to onset, criteria for time of recovery, and list of critical diagnoses to exclude. These issues therefore limit its use in assessing hepatotoxicity.[18] NADRPS has also performed poorly compared to RUCAM. In regard to interobserver variability, agreement between observers was achieved in 45% when using NADRPS compared with 72% using RUCAM scale in a study evaluating 225 suspected cases of DILI.[19] NADRPS, compared with RUCAM, was shown to have a lower sensitivity of 54%, specificity of 88%, PPV of 95%, and NPV of 29%. Observers using NADRPS also seem to differ in their use of clinical judgment in evaluating alternative causes as a diagnosis that critics attribute to lack of standardized methodology within the scale. NADRPS also lacks strict chronologic criteria with respect to the type of liver injury.

DIGESTIVE DISEASE WEEK JAPAN SCALE

The Digestive Disease Week Japan Scale (DDW-J) was derived from the RUCAM scale and proposed in 2004. The scale makes modifications in the items concerning chronologic criteria, use of concomitant drugs, and extrahepatic manifestations that would otherwise suggest hypersensitivity.[4] The DDW-J scale also includes an in vitro drug lymphocyte stimulation test (DLST) as a diagnostic factor that has not been included in other CAMs. When comparing the performance of DDW-J with that of other CAMs, in an analysis of 127 Japanese patients, DDW-J was reported to have a higher sensitivity and a lower specificity (93.8% and 89.1%, respectively) than the RUCAM scale (77.8% and 100%).[20] DDW-J was able to accurately diagnose DILI in some cases that were overlooked using the RUCAM scale. The distribution of cases into probability categories according to the DDW-J scale also indicated higher probability rates than those derived using the RUCAM and M&V scales. In the same study of 127 Japanese patients by Watnabe and Shibuya,[20] the percentage of drugs judged to be "probable" or "highly probable" in the case group was 91.4% using the DDW-J scale compared with 54.7% using the RUCAM scale. Of interest, poor correlation was seen between the two scales despite DDW-J scale representing a modification of the RUCAM scale.

DLST and eosinophilia, included in the DDW-J scale as allergic reactions, are considered to be relevant to DILI. In DDW-J, extrahepatic manifestations suggesting hypersensitivity were evaluated using the DLST (drug lymphocyte stimulation test and rechallenge testing) and from the presence of eosinophilia.[20] The DLST is performed by collecting lymphocytes from heparinized peripheral blood samples of patients. The lymphocytes are then incubated with varying concentrations of the suspected causative drug for 72 hours. Lymphocyte proliferative response is then evaluated by monitoring radiolabeled ^{3}H-thymidine uptake.[17]

In a study by Watanabe and colleagues examining the validity of the DDW-J scale, including DLST and omitting the item of concomitant drug converted nine patients to DILI who were not considered so using the RUCAM scale.[20] By including eosinophilia and omitting the item of concomitant drug, an additional 4 more patients were converted to DILI who were otherwise underestimated by the RUCAM scale.

The investigators concluded that these items seem to improve the sensitivity of DDW-J scale. It was also noted, however, that including DLST and eosinophilia appeared to decrease the specificity of the DDW-J scale. It is known that DLST is sometimes reported as falsely positive and lymphocyte response to the suspected causative drug may not necessarily be related to liver injury.[17,21] Eosinophilia can also be observed in other forms of liver disease.[20] DLST may be useful when a single causative agent cannot be determined (use of concomitant drug use) in select cases.[17] The DDW-J scale may have advantages over the RUCAM and the M&V scales in the diagnosis of DILI. Limited access and lack of standardization have prevented generalized clinical use of the DLST outside Japan and consequently the application of the DDW-J scale.[4] Large-scale statistical evaluations of individual parameters still need to be done in non-Japanese patient populations.

EXPERT OPINION AND THE DRUG-INDUCED LIVER INJURY NETWORK

The diagnostic approach for causality assessment in DILI involves clinical, biochemical, and histologic evaluation, an attempt to establish the latency between the start of drug and the onset of injury, a particular drug or toxin's clinical signature, exclusion of other causes of liver injury, evidence of improvement in the liver injury on dechallenge (drug withdrawal), and possible worsening on rechallenge. When this process is done by an experienced clinician, the evaluation is considered an expert opinion.[22] In the expert opinion process the accessor frames his/her opinion based on personal experiences and general items but without standardized definitions and scores of key elements.

Expert opinion relies on professional opinions on causality after considering all available and relevant data.[4] The qualification of the expert accessor is crucial. Even with specialists, individual opinion often results in judgment differences.[23] Clinical judgment is the cornerstone of the expert opinion method. As a result, this approach is inherently subjective. Furthermore, in cases of several suspected products, expert opinion does not specify the reasons for which one product is the most likely cause. Some studies have shown greater specificity with expert opinion compared with several other algorithms.[24] However, CAMs such as RUCAM were created in part to improve the objective nature of causality assessment and provide a more standardized, less subjective approach.

The most detailed and standardized expert opinion method is used by The US Drug-Induced Liver Injury Network (DILIN). The DILIN was started in 2004 and includes several large referral centers. The network was created to provide a well-characterized and prospectively followed group of patients with DILI on which diagnostic, epidemiologic, and mechanistic studies are done.[22,25] For the assessment of causality, a highly structured expert opinion (SEO) method was developed. The SEO attempts to minimize individual biases and interrater variability by producing a consensus from 3 expert opinions. The SEO method used by the DILIN entails an analysis of a condensed narrative summary consisting of clinical findings, date of onset of liver injury, all medications taken within 6 months of onset of the event, presence of symptoms/signs of liver disease, serial biochemical abnormalities, liver biopsy results if available, and data regarding evaluation for competing causes of liver disease. Additional information provided includes time to improvement or recovery, past use of the implicated agent, concomitant drugs, history of hepatic decompensation or organ failure, and death or liver transplantation.[22]

All reviewers in the SEO method are hepatologists with experience in evaluating DILI. Three independent reviewers grade the likelihood of a causal relationship between the drug and liver injury by 1 of 5 scores (defined as a percentage and descriptively): definite (>95%), highly likely (75%–95%), probable (50%–74%), possible (25%–49%), or unlikely (<25%).[22] A cited strength of the SEO method used in the DILIN is its use of consensus. If all 3 reviewers reach a consensus, meaning they agree on the same causality score independently, this is accepted as the final result. If there is a discrepancy, the chair of the committee attempts to reconcile the differences among them. Failing to find consensus, the full causality committee votes on the case and the causality score with the most votes is accepted as the final score.[22]

The DILIN assessed 250 cases of DILI with both the SEO and RUCAM. Each expert reviewer, using a 5-point category scale, provided an assessment of the likelihood that the medication caused the liver injury and they also completed an RUCAM form. The study found that RUCAM was more conservative in assigning a high level of causality than the DILIN strategy. The DILIN expert opinion process was more likely than RUCAM to ascribe the case to DILI (88.9% vs 63.2%).[22] With the SEO, all 3 reviewers agreed completely in 50 of the cases (27%). In contrast, when RUCAM was used, complete agreement was lower at 19%. This may have been because of the ambiguities of some of the RUCAM score parameters.[22]

The strength of the SEO method is its use of consensus, which is thought to improve reliability. When 100 cases were chosen for retesting with the DILIN SEO method, 73% of reviewers came to the same consensus score on retest and 25% differed by one category. RUCAM was found to have poor reproducibility even when repeated by the same reviewers.[22] The DILIN also notes that consensus prevents one outlier expert opinion from controlling the assessment and therefore helps limit bias. Limitations of the DILIN method include its inherent subjectivity even in the hands of highly experienced clinician investigators. In daily clinical practice, there will be an absence of an expert, which limits the method's widespread applicability. The process is also done retrospectively and can be time consuming and costly, which makes it inaccessible to the clinician needing causality assessment in real time.

DISCUSSION

In that there is no specific objective marker for DILI, accurate and specific causality assessment is challenging. Because of heterogenous DILI symptoms and variability among drugs, it is unlikely that a single unique assessment would fit all forms of presentation. Both reproducibility and validity are required for a causality assessment method. Reproducibility ensures that when comparing results different users arrive at the same assessment despite differences in time and place, whereas validity implies the method is able to distinguish between cases that are related to the drug and those that are not. Without a true gold standard for DILI diagnosis, validity cannot be assessed for any current diagnostic method. Only comparisons between methods can be done, some of which have been summarized in this article.

The challenge in the causality assessment of DILI is that DILI can mimic any liver disease.[20] The diagnosis continues to rely largely on clinical acumen. Many physicians still make a diagnosis of DILI based on their own judgment likely because of the complexity of the scoring systems available.[17] The limitation of clinical experience is the rarity of DILI for the clinician who does not specialize in DILI or liver disease. Causality assessment methods are limited by their inability to prove the connection between a drug and a DILI event.[26] CAM methods, including expert opinion, incorporate rechallenge. However, rechallenge is typically not performed because of risk of severe liver injury and substantial harm to the patient. When rechallenge occurs inadvertently, the response

Table 1
Summary of the most frequently used causality assessment scales[1]

RUCAM Criteria	Score	DDW-J Criteria	Score	NADRPS Criteria	Score	M&V Criteria	Score
Time from drug intake until onset	+1 to +2	Time from drug intake until onset	+1 to +2	Previous reports on this reaction	0 to +1	Time from drug intake until onset	+1 to +3
Time from drug withdrawal until onset	0 to +1	Time from drug withdrawal until onset	0 to +1	Onset of adverse event after the drug was administered	−1 to +2	Time from drug withdrawal until onset	−3 to +3
Course of the reaction	−2 to +3	Course of the reaction	−2 to +3	Dechallenge	0 to +1	Course of the reaction	0 to +3
Risk factors	0 to +2	Risk factors	0 to +1	Rechallenge	−1 to +2	Exclusion of other causes	−3 to +3
Concomitant therapy	−3 to 0	Exclusion of other causes	−3 to +2	Exclusion of alternative causes	−1 to +2	Extrahepatic manifestations	0 to +3
Exclusion of other causes	−3 to +2	Previous information	0 to +1	Reaction with placebo	−1 to +1	Rechallenge	+3
Previous information	−3 to +2	Rechallenge	0 to +3	Drug detected in blood or other fluids in toxic concentrations	0 to +1	Known reaction	−3 to +2
Rechallenge	−2 to +3	Extrahepatic manifestations	0 to +1	Severity of reaction with dose increase or decrease	0 to +1		
		DLST	0 to +2	Prior reactions to the same or similar drugs in any previous exposures?	0 to +1		
				Was the adverse event confirmed by any objective evidence?	0 to +1		

Scores:
>8 points definite
6–8 points probable
3–5 points possible
1–2 points unlikely
<0 points excluded

Scores:
>4 points definite
3–4 points probable
<3 points unlikely

Scores:
≥9 definite
5–8 probable
1–4 possible
≤0 doubtful

Scores:
>17 points definite
14–17 points probable
10–13 points possible
6–9 points unlikely
<6 points excluded

Adapted from Garcia-Cortes M, Stephens C, Lucena MI, Fernandez-Castaner A, Andrade RJ. Causality assessment methods in drug induced liver injury: strengths and weaknesses. *Journal of hepatology.* 2011;55(3):683-691; with permission.

to rechallenge is often unclear, that is, time of assessment after challenge, duration, and dose of rechallenge, and the frequency and timing of testing are not well defined. As a diagnostic test, in and of itself, rechallenge runs the risk of being falsely negative in metabolic and idiosyncratic reactions.[20]

There continues to be research and emerging data regarding potential DILI biomarkers. For example, mircroRNA-122 is a hepatocyte-specific miRNA that is elevated in the plasma of patients within hours of acetaminophen overdose. Although microRNA-122 is liver specific, it is not specific to DILI, which is a recurrent problem encountered in the development of appropriate DILI biomarkers. Hyperacetylated total high-mobility group box protein 1 (HMGB1) is released from immune cells and acts like a marker for immune activation and has been studied in acetaminophen DILI as well as idiosyncratic DILI. The challenge in using HMGB1 is the requirement for mass spectrometry to detect acetylation. Both microRNA-122 and HMGB1 are not drug/toxin specific and have limited use in the currently available CAMs. An ideal biomarker would not only be specific to DILI but would also identify the offending drug or, at a minimum, the class of chemical entities.[26] The identification of ideal biomarkers will continue to be challenging due to the number of potential hepatotoxins, multiple pathogenic mechanisms, and the variable predisposition of patients to DILI.[26]

Certain drugs causing idiosyncratic DILI are associated with the formation of serum autoantibodies. Examples include anti-epoxide hydrolase in germander-induced liver injury, anti-CYP1A2 in dihydralazine hepatitis, anti-CYP3A in anticonvulsant hepatitis, and anti-CYP2E1 in halothane hepatitis.[27] Most experts agree that genetic variations are significant risk factors for DILI.[28] Recent findings of specific human leukocyte antigen (HLA) allele associations with DILI suggest an important role for the adaptive immune response in DILI.[29] Associations have been found between DILI and several HLA genotypes, both class I and II. Studies have shown, for example, that presence of HLA alleles B*5701, DRB1*0701, and DRB1*1501 are associated with flucloxacillin, ximelagatran, and augmentin hepatotoxicity.[28] The use of biomarkers, serum autoantibodies, and genetic variations is yet to be incorporated into causality assessment or clinical practice as standards for diagnosis.

A comparison of the components and corresponding score allocations in the four most commonly used causality assessment scales is shown in **Table 1**. Future directions of causality assessment may also include incorporation of a drug's/toxin's known characteristic clinical, pathologic, and latency presentation into a CAM. This may especially be useful in the setting of concomitant drug exposure; however, the signature presentation of a given drug can vary. More research is also needed regarding the contribution of ethnicity, gender, diabetes, metabolic syndrome, or body mass index and underlying liver disease in DILI causality. Clinicians would benefit from a simplified CAM scoring system with appropriate weighting given to individual parameters that is inclusive of risk factors, biomarkers, and genetic information and is precise in its evaluation of causality and limits ambiguity.[22] Ultimately, DILI causality assessment remains challenging for clinicians; however, the future holds the potential for the development of better algorithms, diagnostic tools, and markers of DILI.

REFERENCES

1. Andrade RJ, Lucena MI, Kaplowitz N, et al. Outcome of acute idiosyncratic drug-induced liver injury: long-term follow-up in a hepatotoxicity registry. Hepatology 2006;44(6):1581–8.

2. National Institutes of Health. Causality. Available at: https://livertox.nih.gov/Causality.html. Accessed March 1, 2019.

3. Das S, Behera SK, Xavier AS, et al. Agreement among different scales for causality assessment in drug-induced liver injury. Clin Drug Investig 2018;38(3):211–8.
4. Garcia-Cortes M, Stephens C, Lucena MI, et al. Causality assessment methods in drug induced liver injury: strengths and weaknesses. J Hepatol 2011;55(3):683–91.
5. Health NIo. RUCAM in DILI. Available at: https://livertox.nih.gov/rucam.html. Accessed March 3, 2019.
6. Hutchinson TA, Lane DA. Assessing methods for causality assessment of suspected adverse drug reactions. J Clin Epidemiol 1989;42(1):5–16.
7. Benichou C, Danan G, Flahault A. Causality assessment of adverse reactions to drugs–II. An original model for validation of drug causality assessment methods: case reports with positive rechallenge. J Clin Epidemiol 1993;46(11):1331–6.
8. Danan G, Benichou C. Causality assessment of adverse reactions to drugs–I. A novel method based on the conclusions of international consensus meetings: application to drug-induced liver injuries. J Clin Epidemiol 1993;46(11):1323–30.
9. Danan G, Teschke R. Drug-induced liver injury: why is the Roussel Uclaf causality assessment method (RUCAM) still used 25 years after its launch? Drug Saf 2018;41(8):735–43.
10. Teschke R, Eickhoff A. The Honolulu liver disease cluster at the medical center: its mysteries and challenges. Int J Mol Sci 2016;17(4):476.
11. Lucena MI, Camargo R, Andrade RJ, et al. Comparison of two clinical scales for causality assessment in hepatotoxicity. Hepatology 2001;33(1):123–30.
12. Larrey D. Epidemiology and individual susceptibility to adverse drug reactions affecting the liver. Semin Liver Dis 2002;22(2):145–55.
13. Kleiner DE. The pathology of drug-induced liver injury. Semin Liver Dis 2009;29(4):364–72.
14. Lucena MI, Andrade RJ, Kaplowitz N, et al. Phenotypic characterization of idiosyncratic drug-induced liver injury: the influence of age and sex. Hepatology 2009;49(6):2001–9.
15. Health NIo. Maria and Victorino (M&V) system of causality assessment in drug induced liver injury. Available at: https://livertox.nih.gov/MVcausality.html. Accessed March 4, 2019.
16. Maria VA, Victorino RM. Development and validation of a clinical scale for the diagnosis of drug-induced hepatitis. Hepatology 1997;26(3):664–9.
17. Tajiri K, Shimizu Y. Practical guidelines for diagnosis and early management of drug-induced liver injury. World J Gastroenterol 2008;14(44):6774–85.
18. Health NIo. Adverse drug reaction probability scale (Naranjo) in drug induced liver injury. Available at: https://livertox.nih.gov/Narajo.html. Accessed March 3, 2019.
19. Garcia-Cortes M, Lucena MI, Pachkoria K, et al. Evaluation of naranjo adverse drug reactions probability scale in causality assessment of drug-induced liver injury. Aliment Pharmacol Ther 2008;27(9):780–9.
20. Watanabe M, Shibuya A. Validity study of a new diagnostic scale for drug-induced liver injury in Japan-comparison with two previous scales. Hepatol Res 2004;30(3):148–54.
21. Maria VA, Pinto L, Victorino RM. Lymphocyte reactivity to ex-vivo drug antigens in drug-induced hepatitis. J Hepatol 1994;21(2):151–8.
22. Rockey DC, Seeff LB, Rochon J, et al. Causality assessment in drug-induced liver injury using a structured expert opinion process: comparison to the Roussel-Uclaf causality assessment method. Hepatology 2010;51(6):2117–26.

23. Teschke R, Eickhoff A, Schulze J. Drug- and herb-induced liver injury in clinical and translational hepatology: causality assessment methods, quo vadis? J Clin Transl Hepatol 2013;1(1):59–74.
24. Macedo AF, Marques FB, Ribeiro CF. Can decisional algorithms replace global introspection in the individual causality assessment of spontaneously reported ADRs? Drug Saf 2006;29(8):697–702.
25. Hayashi PH. Drug-induced liver injury network causality assessment: criteria and experience in the United States. Int J Mol Sci 2016;17(2):201.
26. Teschke R, Schulze J, Eickhoff A, et al. Drug induced liver injury: can biomarkers assist RUCAM in causality assessment? Int J Mol Sci 2017;18(4) [pii:E803].
27. Kullak-Ublick GA, Andrade RJ, Merz M, et al. Drug-induced liver injury: recent advances in diagnosis and risk assessment. Gut 2017;66(6):1154–64.
28. Andrade RJ, Robles M, Ulzurrun E, et al. Drug-induced liver injury: insights from genetic studies. Pharmacogenomics 2009;10(9):1467–87.
29. Stephens C, Lopez-Nevot MA, Lucena MI, et al. 1137 the HLA class I B*1801 allele influences hepatocellular expression of amoxicillin-clavulanate liver damage and outcome IN Spanish patients. J Hepatol 2010;52:S439.

Frequent Offenders and Patterns of Injury

Jinyu Zhang, MD, Deepak Venkat, MD*

KEYWORDS

- DILI • Antimicrobials • Antiepileptics • Immunotherapies • Amiodarone

KEY POINTS

- Antimicrobials account for nearly all of the top 10 causes of DILI published by the DILI Network Group.
- In this article, we focus on commonly used antimicrobials and their patterns of injury.
- Other commonly used drugs discussed in this article include antiepileptics, immunosuppressants, and amiodarone.
- Patterns of injury acutely range from self-limited asymptomatic hepatocellular, cholestatic, or mixed injury to cases of acute liver failure associated with mortality in the absence of transplant.
- Chronic injury patterns again range from asymptomatic elevation in liver function tests to development of chronic cholestatic liver disease, including vanishing bile duct syndrome, autoimmunelike liver disease, and progressive fibrosis with the development of cirrhosis in rare cases.

INTRODUCTION

Given the liver's role in drug metabolism, it is uniquely sensitive to potential drug-induced liver injury (DILI) despite inherent protective mechanisms. In this article, we focus on the most common causes of DILI and their patterns of injury except for analgesics, statins, and drugs/herbal supplements, which are covered in other articles in this issue.

Most cases have distinctive clinical presentations/patterns of injury. Acute injury can present with a hepatocellular (mainly elevations in aminotransferases), cholestatic (mainly elevations in alkaline phosphatase), or mixed pattern of liver enzyme elevation with or without accompanying jaundice and synthetic liver dysfunction. Severity ranges from self-limited mild hepatitis to acute liver failure with high mortality in the absence of emergent liver transplantation. Chronic injury can also take on many forms,

Disclosure Statement: The authors having nothing to disclose.
Division of Gastroenterology and Hepatology, Department of Medicine, Henry Ford Hospital, 2799 West Grand Boulevard K-7, Detroit, MI 48202, USA
* Corresponding author.
E-mail address: Dvenkat1@hfhs.org

Clin Liver Dis 24 (2020) 37–48
https://doi.org/10.1016/j.cld.2019.09.002
1089-3261/20/© 2019 Elsevier Inc. All rights reserved.

liver.theclinics.com

including the development of vanishing bile duct syndrome with progressive chole-stasis and accompanying histologic loss of small intrahepatic bile ducts, chronic autoimmune–like hepatitis, and steatosis or fibrosis with or without accompanying hepatitis.

Although not comprehensive, we attempt to cover several classes of commonly used drugs, and their associated patterns of injury and management.

ANTIMICROBIALS

Antimicrobials, because of their frequency of use, are among the leading causes of DILI and in fact account for nearly all of the top 10 causes of DILI found in a recent review published by the DILI Network group in 2015. In the following sections we cover several antibiotics associated with DILI.

Amoxicillin/Clavulanate

Amoxicillin/clavulanate (Augmentin) is one of the most commonly prescribed antibi-otics, particularly for head and neck and upper respiratory tract infections, with nearly 5 million prescriptions filled annually in the United States. It is the leading cause of DILI in the Western world. The incidence of hepatotoxicity with amoxicillin/clavulanate ranges from 1 to 17 per 100,000 prescriptions.[1] Timing of injury can range from within a few days of starting therapy to several months after completion of therapy with an average of approximately 3 weeks from drug initiation. This most often occurs shortly after completion of the antibiotic course. Because of potential delay in onset, the diag-nosis can be easily missed without thorough history taking. The reaction is idiosyn-cratic in nature.

Clinically, patients can present with nonspecific symptoms including jaundice, nausea, pyrexia, and fatigue. Laboratory abnormalities are typically cholestatic with elevation in alkaline phosphatase and bilirubin, although there have been cases with a mixed and predominantly hepatocellular pattern of injury. A recent study that evaluated more than 100 patients with amoxicillin-clavulanate DILI found that injury was more frequent in men than women (62% vs 39%) with a mean time to symptom onset of approximately 31 days. Resolution of symptoms took approximately 55 days after the peak total bilirubin.[2] Older age has also been implicated as a risk factor for developing DILI.[1] Studies also have shown that HLA Class I and II small nucleotide polymorphisms (SNPs), particularly the SNPs rs9274407, rs9267992, rs3135388, and rs2523822, were associated with amoxicillin-clavulanate DILI.[3] However, this may not be of clinical significance at the current time, as routine testing is not recom-mended before prescription, given loose association with hepatotoxicity, lack of cost-effectiveness, and availability of testing.

Drug withdrawal is the first step in treatment. Recovery can be prolonged after drug cessation ranging from 1 to 6 months and associated with protracted jaundice.[4] Given that the mechanism of injury is thought to be related to an immunoallergic process, with biopsies showing eosinophilia, corticosteroids have been used to accelerate re-covery.[1] However, this is not the standard of care and patients typically recover with drug cessation and supportive care alone.[4]

A minor number of patients do go on to develop acute liver failure.[5] Although a rare event, amoxicillin/clavulanate can also cause chronic liver disease in the form of van-ishing bile duct syndrome characterized by profound and prolonged cholestatic liver injury with accompanying loss of small intrahepatic bile ducts histologically.[6] As such, amoxicillin/clavulanate has been implicated as one of the top causes of chronic DILI. Patients with underlying chronic liver diseases like hepatitis C or fatty liver disease are more likely to develop chronic injury related to amoxicillin/clavulanate; however, underlying chronic liver disease is not a contraindication to its use.[7] Patients may be able to tolerate amoxicillin in the future, as clavulanate is typically felt to be the culprit. Future use of amoxicillin/clavulanate is generally not recommended after an episode of associated DILI; however, use of other beta lactams, including tazobactam, is felt to be safe, as this is not felt to be a class effect.[4]

Isoniazid

INH (Isoniazid) is commonly used as part of an antituberculosis regimen. Despite low prevalence of tuberculosis in the United States, INH is still a leading cause of idiosyncratic DILI. INH-induced hepatotoxicity ranges from mild self-limited elevation in aminotransferase levels to a more severe acute hepatitis with accompanying liver failure. In fact, up to 20% of INH users will experience transient asymptomatic aminotransferase increase,[4] which may spontaneously resolve despite continuation of therapy.

In severe acute injury, patients can present with nonspecific symptoms including fatigue, nausea, and anorexia followed by jaundice. Timing of injury can range from as short as 1 week after starting INH to more than a year after initiation. Pattern of injury is typically more hepatocellular with alanine aminotransferase (ALT) elevations greater than 10 times the upper limit of normal with minimal rise in alkaline phosphatase. There is also an association with antinuclear antibody (ANA) positivity; however, titers are typically low and immunoallergic features do not accompany ANA positivity histologically. Most cases self-resolve; however, approximately 1% of cases of hepatotoxicity may progress to liver failure with up to 0.1% being fatal.[4] In the Acute Liver Failure Group study, INH was the most commonly implicated agent for DILI-induced acute liver failure,[5] and there are several cases that required emergency liver transplantation.

Hepatotoxicity related to INH increases with risk factors such as age (strongest risk factor particularly in those >50), alcohol use or other chronic liver disease, concurrent usage of other medications that induce cytochrome P, prior INH intolerance, African American race, and female gender. Given these risk factors, patients older than 50 or those with underlying chronic liver disease are recommended to have monthly monitoring of liver function tests during INH therapy. It has been proposed by in vitro studies that the Sirtuin 1/Farnesoid X Receptor pathway, as well as downregulation of bile salt export pump and multidrug resistance protein 2 play important roles in INH-induced hepatotoxicity.[4,8] These findings can be seen in several different chronic liver diseases, particularly in those with cirrhosis and as such INH is one of the few medications in which underlying chronic liver disease predicts an increased risk for hepatotoxicity; however, chronic liver disease is not a contraindication to its use.

Current recommendations suggest continued use of INH as long as ALT remains less than 5 times the upper limit of normal. However, should there be any symptoms (eg, anorexia, nausea, jaundice, fatigue) and persistent elevation in aminotransferases more than 3 times the upper limit of normal; temporary cessation of INH therapy is recommended. Rechallenge can be considered on resolution of acute injury, but only in those in whom INH is absolutely required and only with very close monitoring of liver enzymes. There are no clear cutoffs as to when INH must be permanently discontinued, but it has been proposed if a bilirubin of 3 mg/dL and/or liver enzymes more than 5 times the upper limit of normal is ever reached.[9] Steroids have few supporting data in acute injury and are not recommended. There are limited data to support the use of N-acetylcysteine with acute injury; however, most cases resolve with drug cessation and supportive care alone.

Nitrofurantoin

Nitrofurantoin is a commonly prescribed antibiotic for urinary tract infections, whether acutely for treatment or chronically for prophylactic purposes. Liver injury runs the gamut from acute granulomatous reactions and autoimmune-mediated hepatitis to chronic low-grade hepatitis. Overall, risk factors for developing nitrofurantoin-associated hepatotoxicity include older age, chronic long-term use, female sex, and reduced kidney function. Liver injury is idiosyncratic.[4]

The timing of acute injury is typically 1 to 6 weeks after completing a short course of therapy. It is more common in female patients. Pattern of injury is usually hepatocellular and may be accompanied by systemic symptoms (eg, fevers, rash, eosinophilia). Occurrence of jaundice is variable. Acute injury typically subsides quickly after drug cessation alone but acute liver failure can arise.[5] Occasionally, autoimmune features may be seen on biopsy prompting the use of steroids but in most cases of acute injury this is not necessary.

Chronic injury is more common than acute DILI, often presents several months to years into long-term prophylactic therapy, and almost exclusively occurs in female patients. Although the typical injury is that of chronic mild to moderate hepatitis with a hepatocellular pattern of injury, both acute hepatitis with accompanying acute liver failure as well as the rare occurrence of cirrhosis have been reported in those on chronic suppressive therapy. Presentation is often unrecognized, as symptoms occur later in presentation, including jaundice, anorexia, and fatigue. The injury is often autoimmunelike in nature, with elevations in immunoglobulin and presence of autoantibodies including smooth muscle antibody in high titers.[10] However, fever and rash occur less commonly in patients with chronic injury than acute injury. In the DILI Network, of the 60 patients with latency (onset of injury >365 days), nitrofurantoin was found to be the most common drug to be associated with this.[7]

The pathogenesis behind nitrofurantoin-induced liver injury is not clear. Proposals of different mechanisms have suggested a role for CD8+ T-cells, nitroreductive mechanism causing free radical damage to hepatocytes, as well as possible linkage to HLA-DR6/DR2 and HLA-B8/B12.[4,7,9] A prospective study that evaluated nitrofurantoin from the DILI Network (2004–2014) noted that 82% of the nitrofurantoin cases have autoimmune hepatitis–like features. Although the study group was small, n = 29 for nitrofurantoin, the investigators noted that more than two-thirds of the nitrofurantoin cases had some type of ANA and anti-smooth muscle antibody (ASMA) elevation and just under half of them had some immunoglobulin (Ig)G elevation.[11]

On cessation of the drug, complete recovery is typically expected, although may be slow (2–6 months). Due to the autoimmune hepatitis–like features, steroids with rapid taper have been used to treat those with severe presentation or those with slow-to-resolve injury despite drug cessation. Careful follow-up is recommended on steroid withdrawal to monitor for flare.[9] Rechallenge is not recommended, as recurrence of injury is common.

Trimethoprim-Sulfamethoxazole

Trimethoprim-sulfamethoxazole (TMP-SMX) is a common antibiotic used to prevent and treat several commonly occurring and opportunistic infections in both immunocompetent and immunocompromised hosts (human immunodeficiency virus, solid organ transplant recipients).

Liver injury is idiosyncratic and typically accompanied with systemic symptoms of drug-allergy or hypersensitivity, including fevers, rash, and eosinophilia followed by jaundice with days to weeks of starting TMP-SMX. Pattern of injury is typically chole-static, although can be mixed, and less often hepatocellular, although cases of severe acute hepatitis with liver failure have been reported.[4]

Mechanism of injury is thought to relate to an allergic or hypersensitivitylike reaction, most of which has to do with the sulfa component of the drug, but trimethoprim alone also can damage the liver.[4,12] Drug Rash with Eosinophilia and Systemic Symptoms syndrome (DRESS) has been reported with TMP-SMX toxicity with hepatic involve-ment. It also has been reported that granulomatous hepatitis developed due to sulfon-amide hypersensitivity.[13]

Most cases of TMP-SMZ–induced hepatotoxicity are self-limited, with complete re-covery within 2 months of drug cessation.[14] However, patients can progress to acute liver failure or have prolonged cholestasis despite drug withdrawal.[7] Prolonged chole-stasis has been associated with vanishing bile duct syndrome.[6] Recovery from this may take up to 2 years, and some require treatment with ursodeoxycholic acid and anti-pruritogens. Fatality related to TMP/SMZ toxicity is estimated to be 10%.[7] In the DILI Network, TMP-SMZ was one of the top offenders for causing acute liver fail-ure. Because of hypersensitivity, once patients have developed TMP-SMZ DILI, they should avoid future use of this medication, as rechallenge can be associated with acute and severe presentation.[4,7] Steroids may be beneficial in cases associated with fever, rash, and arthralgias or DRESS syndrome.

Minocycline

Minocycline is typically used to treat skin infections and acne. Similarly, certain chemotherapy agents, such as cetuximab and panitumumab, can potentially cause cutaneous skin reactions, therefore minocycline has been used to prevent these reactions.

With minocycline, the incidence of injury is idiosyncratic, and the pattern of injury is generally hepatocellular with 2 types of presentations: an acute severe hepatitis form and a more chronic indolent hepatitis form.[4] In the acute form, patients may present with a viral hepatitis or hypersensitivity-type syndrome, fevers, general malaise, eosin-ophilia, and occasionally atypical lymphocytosis, typically within 1 to 3 months of starting therapy. Patients also may present with exfoliative dermatitis. Liver injury characteristically resolves within 1 to 2 months of stopping therapy. Autoimmune se-rologies can be positive in the acute injury pattern but usually disappear over time.

In the more chronic form, an autoimmune hepatitis–like injury is more common, and can arise years into therapy. The presentation may be that of a severe acute autoim-mune hepatitis flare or that of a smoldering chronic autoimmune–like hepatitis. A pro-spective study that evaluated minocycline from the DILI Network (2004–2014) noted that 73% of the minocycline cases have autoimmune hepatitis–like features. Although the study group was small, n = 19, the investigators noted that more than two-thirds of the cases had some type of ANA elevation, approximately half the cases had ASMA positivity, and approximately one-third of them had some IgG elevation.[11] Most pa-tients do well with cessation of minocycline. Although fibrosis is uncommon, cirrhosis has been related to chronic minocycline use with chronic autoimmune–like features, especially if the drug is continued despite liver function abnormalities. Like nitrofuran-toin, there have been reported cases of using corticosteroids to improve outcomes, although most recover with drug cessation alone.[15] Some experts have argued that if corticosteroids and cessation of drug yield no improvement in transaminitis, to consider azathioprine as a rescue therapy.[16] It also has been noted that in chronic sit-uations, the ANA positivity may persist for a year following cessation of drug.[7] Rechal-lenge is not recommended due to likelihood of recurrence of DILI.

ANTIEPILEPTICS

Seizure and headache disorders are common and as such the use of antiepileptic drugs (AEDs) are common. Several drugs have been associated with the development of hepatotoxicity; however, the most common causes and most severe reactions occur with valproate and phenytoin and are reviewed as follows.

Valproate

Valproate is commonly used to treat seizures, migraines, and mood disorders. Although up to 10% of patients may develop mild increase in liver enzymes on chronic therapy, these abnormalities are usually self-limited even with continuation of the drug; however, there are different forms of clinically relevant DILI that do occur with valproate therapy. Liver injury is typically idiosyncratic and therefore does not necessarily correlate with valproate levels.

The first is a more hepatocellular pattern or mixed form of injury, usually approximately 3 months into therapy.[17] Several cases of fatal acute liver failure have been described due to valproate. Histologically, liver biopsy reveals microvesicular steatosis with central lobular necrosis, with varying degrees of inflammation and fibrosis. In children, valproate has been associated with Reyelike syndrome: fever, lethargy, and microvesicular steatosis on liver biopsy.[4,17] Valproate can cause acute liver failure and is the leading AED-induced acute liver failure requiring transplantation in children.[5,18] Finally, valproate can be associated with a syndrome presenting like hepatic encephalopathy with elevated ammonia levels without abnormal liver function tests or changes on liver biopsy.

The mechanism of hepatic injury associated with valproic acid is thought to be related to damage of mitochondria via decreasing ATP levels and reduction of DNA replication/repair.[19]

It is recommended that once liver enzymes increase to more than 3 times the upper limit of normal, valproate should be discontinued. Mildly abnormal liver enzymes is not a reason to stop therapy. Risk factors associated with more severe reactions include younger age, concurrent therapy with other AEDs, and POLG gene code. Severe hepatotoxicity is rare, estimated to be 1 in 15,000 exposures. Most patients do well with valproate cessation alone. Intravenous carnitine has been used to treat valproate overdose. Experimental data suggest that this L-carnitine could also improve survival in severe valproate-induced hepatotoxicity.[20] Rechallenge is not recommended.

Phenytoin

Phenytoin is commonly used to treat seizures, particularly if they are refractory to other AEDs. It comes in both oral and intravenous (IV) formulations and has been found by the DILI Network to be one of the top IV drug causes of DILI behind antibiotics and antineoplastics.[21]

Like other AEDs, phenytoin can cause asymptomatic elevations in liver enzymes (particularly ALT in the case of phenytoin) without clinical significance. Up to a quarter of those on phenytoin can develop these transient mild elevations in aminotransferase levels and can continue the medication. Black ethnicity is a risk factor for significant phenytoin-induced hepatotoxicity, but the overall calculated risk in the general population is approximately 1 per 10,000 to 50,000 cases.[17]

Most cases of hepatotoxicity are thought to be mediated by a hypersensitivity reaction. Typical symptoms arise within 6 to 8 weeks of therapy. Patients often present with a viral-like syndrome, which may progress into jaundice.[4,22] Pattern of injury varies from hepatocellular, mixed, to cholestatic although it is hypothesized that mixed pattern of injury is more common. Given how commonly minor elevations in ALT are encountered during therapy, routine monitoring after starting is not recommended. Acute hepatitis (ALT >3 times upper limit of normal) with jaundice, however, has a mortality rate of more than 10%. Therefore, if this occurs during therapy, phenytoin should be stopped.[4] DRESS-like syndrome and Steven-Johnson syndrome have been well described in the literature.[5,17] Similar to valproate, phenytoin is one of the more common AEDs to cause acute liver failure leading to liver transplantation listing.[5,18] Once patients develop significant hepatotoxicity related to phenytoin, they should be switched to another AED.[4] In the cases of systemic syndrome associated with toxicity, steroids may have benefit. Cases of chronic injury with vanishing bile duct syndrome have been reported. Rechallenge should be avoided.

IMMUNOTHERAPIES

Autoimmune and immunologic-based disease is widely prevalent; therefore, the use of immunotherapies, particularly in the fields of gastroenterology, rheumatology, and dermatology, are common. Several commonly used drugs can be associated with various patterns of hepatotoxicity, which are summarized as follows.

Methotrexate

Methotrexate is an antimetabolite that is used to treat various diseases: inflammatory bowel disease, psoriasis, rheumatoid arthritis, and hematologic malignancies. Hepatotoxicity is dose dependent and typically associated with aminotransferase elevations rather than cholestatic injury. Both acute and chronic liver injury occur. Acute injury is typically associated with the use of high-dose IV methotrexate. Severe hepatocellular enzyme elevations can occur but usually normalize quickly with cessation of therapy. Chronic injury can take the form of progressive steatosis and fibrosis. Although rare, cases with eventual cirrhosis of the liver can be seen.[4,23] Earlier studies from the 1960s suggest that the prevalence of fibrosis ranges to upward of 50%, whereas cirrhosis ranges to upward of 26%; however, more recent studies note that advanced fibrosis occurs in fewer than 5% of all cases. Older studies are possibly confounded by other risk factors for hepatotoxicity, such as concurrent alcohol use and viral hepatitis.[23] Similarly, modern dosing regimens tend to use much smaller doses of methotrexate and therefore the risk of hepatoxicity and fibrosis is significantly less.

Mechanism of injury is not clear, but thought to be due to activation of Ito cells: when activated in the setting of persistent liver injury, myelofibroblasts form subsequently secreting matrix protein; and persistent depletion of folate, therefore altering DNA synthesis.[23] Methotrexate hepatotoxicity is exacerbated by other risk factors for liver disease, including metabolic syndrome, alcohol use, and other liver diseases, such as hepatitis C or hepatitis B. Folate supplementation possibly mitigates hepatotoxicity. Cumulative dosing also affects methotrexate-induced liver injury. Daily, every other day, or 3 divided doses within a week are associated with a fourfold increase in fibrosis, whereas long-term, low-dose (<20 mg), once-weekly regimen without other risk factors are not associated with an increased risk in fibrosis.[7,24]

Monitoring liver enzymes is recommended when patients are on methotrexate. Currently, the American College of Rheumatology recommends more frequent monitoring (every 4 weeks) when initiating methotrexate with less frequent monitoring as time progresses (every 12 weeks once past 6 months if enzymes remain normal).[25] The National Psoriasis Foundation recommends monitoring of liver enzymes every 4 to 12 weeks and that laboratory tests should be drawn ideally 5 days following methotrexate administration, as liver enzymes may be elevated in the first 1 to 2 days after methotrexate dosing.[26] Rheumatology and dermatology guidelines recommend consideration of dose reduction with any abnormality in liver enzymes with repeat testing in 2 to 4 weeks to ensure normalization or improvement in liver enzymes. Liver biopsy should be considered if aminotransferases were to remain persistently elevated after dose modification or cessation of methotrexate.[27] Liver biopsy also is indicated if there were aminotransferase elevations in 6 blood draws over a 12-month period or if there were to be a significant decline in albumin to exclude progressive fibrosis. In the past, various societies recommend fibrosis assessment once certain cumulative doses of methotrexate are reached (for example after 1, 3, and 8 g cumulative doses). Experts have called this recommendation into question because of the low risk of fibrosis in the absence of abnormal liver enzymes and with modern dosing regimens, but this is controversial and several specialists still prefer monitoring for fibrosis in patients after certain cumulative doses of methotrexate. Pretreatment fibrosis assessment is recommended in patients with other concomitant chronic liver disease (alcohol, nonalcoholic fatty liver, viral hepatitis) to exclude significant pretreatment fibrosis. Similarly, alcohol cessation is recommended before treatment with methotrexate. The gastroenterology associations do not routinely recommend liver biopsies in patients with inflammatory bowel disease (IBD) on methotrexate, as incidence of methotrexate toxicities in patients with IBD tend to be low.[28] The role of elastography as opposed to biopsy for monitoring of fibrosis progression in patients on methotrexate is currently evolving. If patients develop advanced fibrosis or cirrhosis, drug should be permanently discontinued. Cases of hepatitis B reactivation have been reported in patients on both acute high-dose and chronic low-dose methotrexate, particularly in those who are positive for hepatitis B surface antigen (HBSAg). As such, either close monitoring or antiviral prophylaxis is recommended in HBSAg-positive patients receiving methotrexate.

Azathioprine/6-Mercaptopurine

Azathioprine (AZA), a pro-drug of 6-mercaptopurine (6-MP), which inhibits T-cell maturation, was initially developed as an antineoplastic drug, then transitioned to being an anti–transplant rejection medication but over time has been used more so in autoimmune conditions, such as IBD and autoimmune hepatitis. AZA is metabolized to 6-MP, which gets metabolized to 6-MMP (6-methylmercaptopurine) by TPMT (thiopurine methyltransferase); 6-MMP can directly cause hepatotoxicity. It has been hypothesized that although overall low-risk, elevated 6-MMP levels of more than 5700 pmol/8×10^8 red blood cells may be associated with hepatotoxicity.[29]

Hepatotoxicity from thiopurines run the gamut: 4 patterns of injury have been identified. The most common type of injury is a transient, asymptomatic, hepatocellular injury that occurs in fewer than 20% of patients and usually in the first 12 weeks of treatment. Injury is often self-limited and may resolve even with continued administration of AZA. A second form of injury is that of progressive cholestatic injury with minimal elevation in ALT. This usually develops after 2 to 12 months of therapy and can be profound and prolonged, occasionally accompanied by vanishing bile duct syndrome. Other forms of injury, including peliosis hepatis, nodular regenerative hyperplasia, and sinusoidal obstruction syndrome occur after longer periods of therapy (1–5 years) and are felt to be rare.[7,30,31] Liver injury more commonly occurs in women, associated with higher doses of drugs (particularly if >50 mg/d), and clinically presents with nonspecific symptoms. Patients may be anicteric.[30] Underlying liver steatosis has been identified as a risk factor for hepatotoxicity in patients with IBD on thiopurines.[32]

Because of the risk of hepatotoxicity, it is recommended to monitor liver enzymes monthly on initiation of AZA, with less frequent monitoring (every 12 weeks) if no signs of hepatotoxicity are encountered initially.

On cessation of thiopurines, most patients have favorable prognosis. Although rare, a few patients across the DILI Network have undergone liver transplantation for acute liver failure related to thiopurines.[18]

Tumor Necrosis Factor-α Inhibitors

Infliximab, adalimumab, golimumab, certolizumab, and etanercept are TNF-α inhibitors typically used to treat rheumatologic disease as well as IBD. To date, there have been no case reports of golimumab or certolizumab causing significant liver injury, although both drugs can cause asymptomatic transient rise of ALT without clinical significance.[4] Anti-TNF-α therapy is less likely than methotrexate and AZA/6-MP to cause DILI. It is well known that TNF-α inhibitors can lead to reactivation of hepatitis B, and is categorized by American Association for the Study of Liver Diseases guidelines as being moderate risk for hepatitis B reactivation.[33] The Food and Drug Administration approved infliximab in 1998 and issued a hepatotoxic warning on it in 2004; however, incidence was noted to be low, approximately 1 case in every 16,500 treated people.[34,35]

Anti-TNF-α pattern of injury is typically hepatocellular, but can be cholestatic. Less commonly, patients will develop a prolonged cholestatic injury. Most cases of acute hepatocellular injury typically occur approximately 3 months after drug initiation, but latency more than 6 months can occur; and delayed cases are typically related to an immune-mediated mechanism of injury. In cases of immune-mediated injury, autoimmune markers, ANA, ASMA, anti–double-stranded DNA, can be elevated. Liver biopsies show changes consistent with autoimmune hepatitis: interface hepatitis, plasma cells, and piecemeal necrosis. Direct hepatocellular toxicity rather than autoimmunelike injury is less common. Liver biopsy shows intralobular spotty necrosis with aggregates of hypertrophied, ceroid-containing Kupffer cells, and mononuclear inflammatory cell infiltrate at the portal tract.[4,21,34]

Prognosis on withdrawal of anti-TNF-α is typically good, and steroids are helpful in autoimmunelike cases to accelerate recovery; however, there has been reported a case of nonresponse to steroids requiring subsequent liver transplantation.[21,34] Steroid withdrawal after 3 to 6 months of biochemical remission has been suggested.[36] Despite developing hepatotoxicity related to anti-TNF-α therapy, patients may be successfully switched to another anti-TNF-α without problems. There have been case reports of a patient doing well with adalimumab following infliximab-induced liver injury, as well as successful switch to etanercept following adalimumab-induced liver injury.[37,38] TNF therapy is felt to be moderate risk for hepatitis B reactivation, and as such HBSAg-positive patients should receive antiviral prophylaxis.

CARDIAC DRUGS
Amiodarone

Amiodarone is commonly used to treat cardiac arrythmias. With chronic therapy, the pattern of liver injury associated is typically hepatocellular, but can be cholestatic. Aminotransferases increase in approximately 25% of patients on chronic oral therapy, typically more aspartate aminotransferase than ALT, and will generally disappear despite continued therapy.[39] Most remain asymptomatic. Pattern of injury is like that of alcohol-induced injury with steatosis, Mallory bodies, neutrophilic lobular inflammation, ballooning degeneration, and occasionally varying degrees of fibrosis.[4,7] This is likely due to similar pathophysiology, including direct mitochondrial toxicity. Fewer than 3% of patients will develop significant hepatitis or progression to cirrhosis.

Cardiology practice guidelines recommend checking liver enzymes at baseline and every 6 months; and to discontinue amiodarone should there be a twofold increase in liver enzymes.[40] Studies have suggested that there is a dose-dependent and cumulative effect regarding liver insult, possibly related to the long half-life of amiodarone.[41] As such, recovery from chronic injury may be prolonged even after drug withdrawal.[39] In addition, in vitro studies suggest that a high CYP3A4 activity is a risk factor for hepatototoxicty.[42] Although extremely rare, progression to cirrhosis has been reported in multiple case reports.

A distinct pattern of injury can be seen in patients on IV amiodarone with aminotransferases that can rise 10-fold to 100-fold.[4,43] Although most cases will improve in a few days with drug withdrawal, cases of acute liver failure have been seen.[4] There may be a role for N-acetylcysteine in these cases, although data are limited.[44]

SUMMARY

DILI can present variably due to a wide variety of drugs. Acutely, it may present with hepatocellular, cholestatic, or mixed injury with various clinical phenotypes ranging from mild transient asymptomatic rise in liver enzymes to fulminant liver failure, oftentimes mediated by immunologic or direct toxicity to hepatocytes. Chronically, patients can have a wide variety of presentations from asymptomatic development of steatosis and fibrosis to chronic autoimmune–like hepatitis to cases of vanishing bile duct syndrome following acute injury. Although most patients recover, given that reactions are typically idiosyncratic with underrecognition of the condition, latency in presentations and sometimes continuation of medication despite changes in liver enzymes, cases of liver failure due occur sometimes requiring liver transplantation or resulting in fatality. For most drugs, there are no specific therapies or antidotes besides cessation and supportive care, although in some cases steroids and N-acetylcysteine may have a role.

Although we have covered several classes of drugs and patterns of injury, there are several other medications that can be associated with liver injury. Unfortunately, a comprehensive review is beyond the scope of this article. Several resources are available to clinicians for more detail. A few common themes do emerge on review, however. For one, the incidence of injury is relatively rare even with widely prescribed medications, as such for most medications, routine monitoring of liver enzymes is not recommended. Second, the severity of underlying liver disease typically does not predict a higher risk for hepatotoxicity nor does it represent a contraindication to the use of most medications, although closer monitoring may be warranted in patients with chronic liver disease receiving potentially hepatotoxic medications. Finally, in most cases, rechallenge is not recommended because of the likelihood of recurrent injury.

REFERENCES

1. Herrero-Herrero JI, Garcia-Aparicio J. Corticosteroid therapy in a case of severe cholestatic hepatitis associated with amoxicillin-clavulanate. J Med Toxicol 2010; 6(4):420–3.
2. deLemos AS, Ghabril M, Rockey DC, et al. Amoxicillin-clavulanate-induced liver injury. Dig Dis Sci 2016;61(8):2406–16.
3. Lucena MI, Molokhia M, Shen Y, et al. Susceptibility to amoxicillin-clavulanate-induced liver injury is influenced by multiple HLA class I and II alleles. Gastroenterology 2011;141(1):338–47.

4. LiverTox: clinical and research information on drug-induced liver injury. National Institutes of Health. Available at: https://livertox.nlm.nih.gov/. Accessed April 1, 2019.
5. Reuben A, Koch DG, Lee WM. Drug-induced acute liver failure: results of a U.S. multicenter prospective study. Hepatology 2010;52(6):2065–76.
6. Bonkovsky HL, Kleiner DE, Gu J, et al. Clinical presentations and outcomes of bile duct loss caused by drugs and herbal dietary supplements. Hepatology 2017;65(4):1267–77.
7. Stine JG, Chalasani N. Chronic liver injury induced by drugs: a systematic review. Liver Int 2015;35:2343–53.
8. Qu X, Zhang Y, Zhang S, et al. Dysregulation of BSEP and MRP2 may play an important role in isoniazid-induced liver injury via the SIRT1/FXR pathway in rats and HepG2 cells. Biol Pharm Bull 2018;41:1211–8.
9. Badrinath M, John S. Isoniazid toxicity. Florida: StatPearls Publishing; 2018.
10. Sakaan SA, Twilla JD, Usery JB, et al. Nitrofurantoin-induced hepatotoxicity: a rare yet serious complication. South Med J 2014;107(2):107–13.
11. de Boer YS, Kosinski AS, Urban TJ, et al. Features of autoimmune hepatitis in patients with drug-induced liver injury. Clin Gastroenterol Hepatol 2017;15(1):103–12.e2.
12. Mainra RR, Card SE. Trimethroprim-sulfamethoxazole associated hepatotoxicity – part of a hypersensitivity syndrome. Can J Clin Pharmacol 2003;10:175–8.
13. Espiritu CR, Kim TS, Levine RA. Granulomatous hepatitis associated with sulfadimethoxine hypersensitivity. JAMA 1967;202:985–9.
14. Abusin S, Johson S. Sulfamethoxazole/Trimethroprim induced liver failure: a case report. Cases J 2008;1(1):44.
15. Ford TJ, Dillon JF. Minocycline hepatitis. Eur J Gastroenterol Hepatol 2008;20:796–9.
16. Harmon EG, McConnie R, Kesavan A. Minocycline induced autoimmune hepatitis: a rare but important cause of drug-induced autoimmune hepatitis. Pediatr Gastroenterol Hepatol Nutr 2018;21(4):347–50.
17. Vidaurre J, Gedela S, Yarosz S. Antiepileptic drugs and liver disease. Pediatr Neurol 2017;77:23–36.
18. Mindikoglu AL, Magder LS, Regev A. Outcome of liver transplantation for drug-induced acute liver failure in the United States. Analysis of the united network for organ sharing database. Liver Transpl 2009;15(7):719–29.
19. Ramachandran A, Duan L, Akakpo JY, et al. Mitochondrial dysfunction as mechanism of drug-induced hepatotoxicity: current understanding and future perspectives. J Clin Transl Res 2018;4(1):75–100.
20. Lheureux PE, Hantson P. Carnitine in the treatment of valproic acid-induced toxicity. Clin Toxciol (Phila) 2009;47(2):101–11.
21. Ghabril M, Fontana R, Rockey D, et al. Drug-induced liver injury caused by intravenously administered medications: the drug-induced liver injury network experience. J Clin Gastroenterol 2013;47(6):553–8.
22. Smythe MA, Umstead GS. Phenytoin hepatotoxicity: a review of the literature. DICP 1989;23(1):13–8.
23. Bath R, Brar N, Forouhar F, et al. A review of methotrexate-associated hepatotoxicity. J Dig Dis 2014;15(10):517–24.
24. Shetty A, Cho W, Alazawi W, et al. Methotrexate hepatotoxicity and the impact of nonalcoholic fatty liver disease. Am J Med Sci 2017;354(2):172–81.
25. Singh JA, Saag KG, Bridges SL, et al. 2015 American College of Rheumatology Guideline for the treatment of rheumatoid arthritis. Arthritis Care Res 2016;58(1):1–25.

26. Kalb RE, Strober B, Weinstein G, et al. Methotrexate and psoriasis: 2009 National Psoriasis Foundation consensus conference. J Am Acad Dermatol 2009;60(5): 824–37.
27. Busger Op Vollenbroek FTM, Doggen CJM, Janssens RWA, et al. Dermatological guidelines for monitoring methotrexate treatment reduce drug-survival compared to rheumatological guidelines. PLoS One 2018;13(3):e0194401.
28. Herfarth HH, Kappelman MD, Long MD, et al. Use of methotrexate in the treatment of inflammatory bowel diseases (IBD). Inflamm Bowel Dis 2016;22(1): 224–33.
29. Shaye OA, Yadegari M, Abreu MT, et al. Hepatotoxicity of 6-mercaptopurine and azathiopurine in adult IBD patients. Am J Gastroenterol 2007;102:2488–94.
30. Björnsson ES, Gu J, Kleiner DE, et al. Azathioprine and 6-mercaptopurine-induced liver injury: clinical features and outcomes. J Clin Gastroenterol 2017; 51(1):63–9.
31. de Boer NKH, Mulder CJJ, van Bodegrave AA. Myelotoxicity and hepatotoxicity during azathioprine therapy. Neth J Med 2005;63(11):444–6.
32. Schröder T, Schmidt KJ, Olsen V. Liver steatosis is a risk factor for hepatotoxicity in patients with inflammatory bowel disease under immunosuppressive treatment. Eur J Gastroenterol Hepatol 2015;27(6):698–704.
33. Terrault NA, Lok ASF, McMahon BJ, et al. Update on prevention, diagnosis, and treatment of chronic hepatitis B: AASLD 2018 hepatitis B guidance. Hepatology 2018;67(4):1560–99.
34. Mancini S, Amorotti E, Vecchio S, et al. Infliximab-related hepatitis: discussion of a case and review of the literature. Intern Emerg Med 2010;5:193–200.
35. Ghabril M, Bonkovsky HL, Kum C, et al. Liver injury from tumor necrosis factor-α antagonists: analysis of thirty-four cases. Clin Gastroenterol Hepatol 2013;11(5): 558–64.
36. Rodrigues S, Lopes S, Magro F, et al. Autoimmune hepatitis and anti-tumor necrosis factor alpha therapy: a single center report of 8 cases. World J Gastroenterol 2015;21(24):7584–8.
37. Cravo M, Silva R, Serrano M. Autoimmune hepatitis induced by infliximab in a patient with Crohn's disease with no relapse after switching to adalimumab. BioDrugs 2010;24(Suppl 1):25–7.
38. Massarotti M, Marasini B. Successful treatment with etanercept of a patient with psoriatic arthritis after adliumamb-related hepatotoxicity. Int J Immunopathol Pharmacol 2009;22(2):547–9.
39. Lewis JH, Ranard RC, Caruso A, et al. Amiodarone hepatotoxicity: prevalence and clinicopathologic correlations among 104 patients. Hepatology 1989;9(5): 679–85.
40. Goldschlager N, Epstein AE, Naccarelli G, et al. Practical guidelines for clinicians who treat patients with amiodarone. Arch Intern Med 2000;160:1741–8.
41. Vorperian VR, Havighurst TC, Miller S, et al. Adverse effects of low dose amiodarone: a meta-analysis. J Am Coll Cardiol 1997;30(3):791–8.
42. Zahno A, Brecht K, Morand R, et al. The rold of CYP3A4 in amiodarone-associated toxicity on HepG2 cells. Biochem Pharmacol 2001;81(3):432–41.
43. Babatin M, Lee SS, Pollak PT. Amiodarone hepatotoxicity. Curr Vasc Pharmacol 2008;6(3):228–36.
44. Mudadel ML, Dave KP, Hummel JP, et al. N-acetylcysteine treats intravenous amiodarone induced liver injury. World J Gastroenterol 2015;21(9):2816–9.

Quantitative Systems Toxicology Approaches to Understand and Predict Drug-Induced Liver Injury

Paul B. Watkins, MD

KEYWORDS

- DILIsym • DILI • QST • Simulation • Modeling

KEY POINTS

- The DILI-sim Initiative is a public-private partnership that has applied quantitative systems toxicology modeling to develop software (DILIsym®) that has improved mechanistic understanding of DILI.
- DILIsym incorporates pharmacokinetics and ability to alter key hepatocyte pathways to predict the frequency and severity of liver injury by drugs in simulated patient populations.
- Although DILIsym has been largely tested on drugs whose liver safety liability is already established, clinical trials are ongoing that will test its ability to prospectively predict liver safety before clinical trials are conducted.
- DILIsym also has been useful in optimizing interpretation of traditional liver chemistry tests and is incorporating new and promising biomarkers of liver injury.
- With further refinement of DILIsym, its predictions of liver safety may reduce the size of clinical trials required to establish liver safety and also may be useful in the clinic in managing DILI risk.

INTRODUCTION

Quantitative systems toxicology (QST) uses mathematical equations to recapitulate relevant pathways whereby drugs or other chemicals can cause death to cells and organs.[1] The major QST effort currently is focused on drug-induced liver injury (DILI) is the DILI-sim Initiative.[2] This is a public-private partnership established in 2011 to understand and predict the liver safety liability of new drug candidates. It involves

Disclosure: Dr P.B. Watkins chairs the Scientific Advisory Committee for the DILI-sim Initiative and receives compensation for this role. He also has a financial interest in the spinoff company DILIsym Services, Inc, which is a subsidiary of Simulations Plus.
Funding: No funding was received for this work.
Institute for Drug Safety Sciences, Eshelman School of Pharmacy, The University of North Carolina at Chapel Hill, 6 Davis Drive, PO Box 12137, Research Triangle Park, NC 27709, USA
E-mail address: pbwatkins@email.unc.edu

Clin Liver Dis 24 (2020) 49–60
https://doi.org/10.1016/j.cld.2019.09.003
1089-3261/20/© 2019 Elsevier Inc. All rights reserved.

liver.theclinics.com

scientists from academia, the Food and Drug Administration (FDA), and pharmaceutical companies and has funding commitments until at least 2021. Partners in the Initiative vote to prioritize directions for the modeling, assuring that the software addresses the most pressing needs in drug development.

In the DILI-sim Initiative, the pathways whereby drugs can injure the liver are represented using differential equations in submodels, which are connected with the outcome of hepatocyte death and release of biomarkers into serum. **Fig. 1** gives an overview of the submodels. DILIsym is the brand name of the evolving model, which is currently in version 8A. There are mouse, rat, and dog as well as human versions of the model.[3,4] The first drug modeled by the initiative was acetaminophen where oxidative stress could account for toxicity observed with overdose in rodents and man. The modeling was used to propose the optimal protocol for treatment of acetaminophen overdoses with N-acetyl cysteine.[5] The modeling was also then used to evaluate several hypotheses for why the isomer of acetaminophen, 3'-hydroxyacetanilide (AMAP), which also generates reactive metabolites, is much less toxic than acetaminophen in mice.[6]

The continued development of DILIsym has been based on data from many exemplar drugs with varying liver safety profiles, including drugs that had discordant results in preclinical and clinical testing. Exemplar drugs chosen for modeling

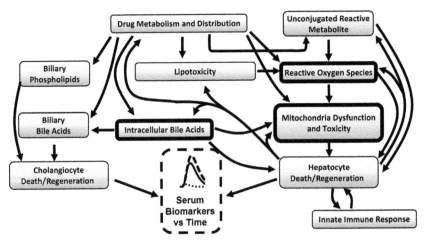

Fig. 1. Submodels in DILIsym. Submodels for hepatocellular injury include production of reactive metabolites, generation of reactive oxygen species (oxidative stress), mitochondrial dysfunction and accumulation of toxic bile acids within the hepatocytes, lipotoxicity, and activation of an innate immune response. These processes are integrated with the potential outcome of hepatocyte death by either apoptosis or necrosis, resulting in different rates of release of traditional and experimental biomarkers into blood. The model also includes some adaptation mechanisms that reduce injury, including Farnesoid X receptor activation by bile acid accumulation, mitochondrial biogenesis initiated by adenosine triphosphate reduction, nuclear factor erythroid 2–related factor 2 response to oxidative stress. Hepatocyte regeneration to compensate for hepatocyte loss is incorporated in the model, and the functioning hepatocyte mass determines global liver function at any point in time. When loss of hepatocyte mass reaches 30%, the predicted serum bilirubin rises due to loss of global liver function. The modeling has suggested that the 3 mechanisms outlined in thick boxes can account for hepatotoxicity in rats and man for more than 80% of the drugs in the validation cohort tested to date. The current version of the model also includes injury to cholangiocytes by inhibiting MDR3-mediated secretion of phospholipids into bile.

have included drugs where relevant data were publicly available and also unpublished data on drugs provided by the industry partners. To recapitulate the known safety profile of each exemplar drug, the model parameters were optimized. Once the model was optimized in this way, the Initiative began testing a new validation set of drugs where the preclinical and clinical safety profiles were known. As of May 2019, 68 molecules have been prospectively tested, with an 80% success in correctly identifying the presence or absence of a liver safety liability at the administered dosing (Brett Howell, personal communication, 2019). Among the 20% failures, all but 1 were predictions of safety with drugs that had exhibited some degree of hepatotoxicity (ie, false negatives).

DATA INPUTS TO DILIsym

The way DILIsym is typically used to assess the liver safety of a drug is illustrated in **Fig. 2**. Physiologically based pharmacokinetic (PBPK) modeling is created using available pharmacokinetic data and other relevant data (eg, liver-to-blood ratio of radioactivity in a rodent mass balance study) to estimate the time-dependent exposure of the drug outside and inside the hepatocyte. If the drug is a known substrate for uptake or efflux transporters, this fact is also taken into consideration in the PBPK model.

The properties of the drug relevant to hepatotoxicity are then assessed with in vitro systems. To screen for hepatocellular DILI potential, the drug is typically tested for its concentration-dependent ability to (1) inhibit bile acid transporters and thereby raise bile acid concentration in hepatocytes, (2) inhibit mitochondrial respiration, and (3) cause oxidative stress. If major metabolites are available, these typically also undergo these assays.

There are multiple hepatocyte transporters that can influence the intrahepatocyte concentration of bile acids,[7] and the ability of a drug to inhibit each of these transporters is typically assayed. Some degree of inhibition of the bile salt export pump (BSEP) seems to be generally required to cause hepatotoxicity based on alterations in bile acid homeostasis, but the additional contribution resulting from inhibition of the basolateral efflux transporters MRP3 and MRP4 can be substantial. Conversely, inhibition of the major bile acid uptake pump, NTCP, would result in lowering of hepatocyte concentration of bile acids. Many drugs that inhibit efflux transporters also inhibit NTCP, creating a complex situation ideal for modeling.

The ability to inhibit mitochondrial respiration and to generate oxidative stress has been typically measured in a human hepatoma cell line, HepG2, using the Seahorse (Agilent Industries, Santa Clara, CA, United States) instrument and high content imaging, respectively. Because lipotoxicity is an infrequent mechanism of DILI, this property is assessed only if suspected. In addition to assessing the effect of the drug as a function of media concentration, the intracellular drug (and metabolite) concentration is also assessed using mass spectroscopy.

When modeling cholangiocyte injury, an assessment is made of the concentration-dependent ability of the drug and metabolites to inhibit a canalicular efflux transporter, multidrug-resistant protein 3 (MDR3). MDR3 transports into bile phospholipids that are incorporated into micelles. There are growing data to support the idea that reduction in biliary phospholipid reduces encapsulation of bile acids in micelles and that the resultant naked bile acids can be toxic to cholangiocytes.[8] Cholangiocyte culture systems are currently being evaluated for the ability to generate relevant data, reflecting direct toxicity of the drug/metabolite to cholangiocytes.

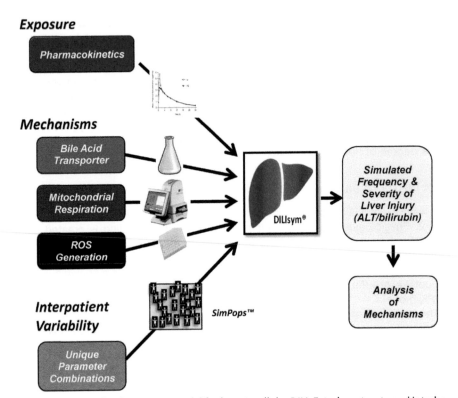

Fig. 2. Data inputs for the DILIsym model for hepatocellular DILI. Extrahepatocyte and intrahepatocyte exposure to study drug is assessed by PBPK modeling and other available data (see text). The dose-dependent effects of drug and major metabolites then are assessed on (1) bile acid transporters expressed in membrane vesicles, cell lines overexpressing transporters, or hepatocytes; (2) mitochondrial respiration in hepatocytes or hepatocyte cell lines using the Seahorse instrument; and (3) reactive oxygen species (ROS) generation measured with high content imaging also in hepatocyte cell lines or primary hepatocytes. The exposure estimates and collected mechanistic data are put into the model, which will then predict the time-dependent death of hepatocytes and hence the time-dependent release of biomarkers (typically ALT) into serum in an average patient. In addition, modeling can be conducted in Simpops® that have been created by changing parameters in the model to capture interpatient variation due to genetic or nongenetic factors. Thus, estimates can be made of the frequency as well as the extent of liver injury in a specific patient population targeted to receive the drug. If a drug causes elevations in liver injury biomarkers, hepatotoxicity can be minimized or eliminated in the Simpops by varying dose and liver chemistry monitoring parameters. This modeling has been helpful in designing clinical trials of new drug candidates (see text). (*From* Watkins PB. The DILI-sim Initiative: Insights into Hepatotoxicity Mechanisms and Biomarker Interpretation. Clinical and translational science. 2019;12(2):122-9; with permission.)

The methods chosen to gather the data necessary for predictive modeling have been chosen by the DILI-sim Initiative partners because these methods are commercially available if not already up and running in their organizations.

Data Outputs from DILIsym

When the compound data collected are input into the model, together with estimates of the time-dependent concentration of the drug and major metabolites outside and inside hepatocytes, the model then predicts the time-dependent death of hepatocytes and hence the time-dependent release of certain biomarkers into serum (see **Fig. 1**). The biomarker of most interest is generally serum alanine aminotransferase (ALT) because this is the most specific and sensitive among traditional biomarkers for hepatocyte death. Time-dependent changes in total bilirubin are also estimated based on the predicted loss of hepatocyte mass. In the model, bilirubin elevations to greater than 2-times the upper limit of normal (ULN) occur when the viable fraction of hepatocytes falls below 70%, a figure based on liver biopsy data obtained from patients experiencing liver injury due to acetaminophen overdose.[9] Experimental biomarkers,[10] including glutamate dehydrogenase, microRNA 122, full-length K18, and the caspase-cleaved fragment of cytokeratin 18, are also data outputs from the model, and incorporation of additional experimental biomarkers is planned.

The simplest output from DILIsym is predictions for an average healthy individual but DILIsym also can display predictions for simulated patient populations. This is done by varying parameters in the model to reflect interpatient variation in response resulting from genetic or nongenetic factors. The simulated populations (Simpops®) include patients with nonalcoholic steatohepatitis (NASH) and diabetes. Where possible, the model parameters for the patient-specific populations are varied based on experimental data, such as the reduction in activity in enzymes involved in mitochondrial oxidative phosphorylation observed in liver biopsies obtained from patients with NASH.[11] Other parameters have been varied to fit data obtained from clinical trials involving the specific patient populations. New Simpops are planned for other patient populations, including children.

In addition to graphs for predicted liver chemistries over time, DILIsym can display predictions in evaluation of drug-induced serious hepatotoxicity (eDISH) format.[12] eDISH is now a standard way the FDA evaluates liver safety of new drug candidates, generally from data obtained in phase 3 clinical trials. eDISH creates a graph, where, for each subject in a clinical trial, the observed peak serum ALT value is plotted along the X-axis and the observed peak serum bilirubin value along the Y-axis (ie, each subject is represented by a single point on the graph). Examples of eDISH graphs predicted by DILIsym are shown in **Fig. 3**. In this case, the modeling predicted that liver injuries, including severe liver injuries (ie, Hy's law cases), would be encountered at high daily doses of the modeled drug. Safe dosing regimens, however, could be predicted.

Identifying Dominant Mechanisms Underlying Drug-Induced Liver Injury

Once liver safety liability of a drug is predicted by DILIsym, it is possible to identify which of the 3 mechanisms is contributing most to the predicted toxicity. This is done by simply turning off each mechanism in the model, 1 at a time, and observing the effect this has on the predicted frequency of serum ALT elevations in the Simpops. Typically, no 1 mechanism accounts for the predicted toxicity and there are instances where at least 2 mechanisms must be operative to produce any toxicity.[13] There are as yet unpublished examples of where identifying the major mechanism underlying the toxicity of a drug has explained drug-drug interactions associated with increased frequency of elevations in serum ALT in clinical trials (Brett Howell, personal communication).

The prominence of the 3 mechanisms in accounting for toxicity is remarkable because none directly takes into account some DILI mechanisms that generally are recognized to be important, such as reactive metabolite production[14] and endoplasmic reticulum stress.[15] Such mechanisms may account for the approximately 20% failure rate of the current model predictions and addition of new mechanisms

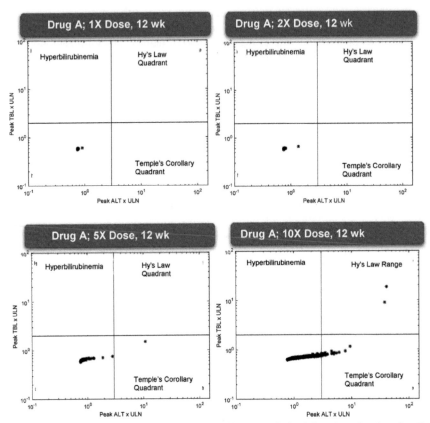

Fig. 3. eDISH output from DILIsym modeling of hepatocellular injury in a simulated patient population treated with drug A. eDISH is the method typically used to assess liver safety in large clinical trials. Each dot represents a subject in the clinical trial and the location of the dot on the eDISH plot corresponds to the peak serum ALT (X-axis) and total serum bilirubin (Y-axis) observed in that subject. The graph is divided into 5 quadrants by a vertical line at the value of 3-times the ULN for ALT and a horizontal line at the value of 2-times the ULN for bilirubin. At the modeled 1-times the dose daily for 12 weeks, no simulated patients experienced a rise in serum ALT (the *dots* correspond to <1-times the ULN [10^0]). At 2-times the dose, 1 simulated subject experienced a rise in serum ALT greater than ULN but less than 3-times the ULN. At 5-times the dose, several simulated subjects experienced ALT elevations, and 1 subject reached greater than 3-times the ULN. This subject did not experience global liver dysfunction sufficient to result in an elevation in serum total bilirubin greater than 2-times the ULN and subject's point, therefore, appears in the right lower quadrant (also call Temple's corollary quadrant). At the 10-times dose, however, 2 simulated patients appear in the right upper quadrant (Hy's law quadrant) indicating sufficient loss of hepatocytes to cause global liver dysfunction. TBIL, total bilirubin.

to DILIsym is likely in the future. It also is possible that there exist correlations with the mechanisms in the model such that those left out are indirectly taken into account. For example, a reactive metabolite may produce oxidative stress and oxidative stress can result in endoplasmic reticulum stress. Parent and major metabolites have been routinely tested in a human hepatoma cell line (Hep G2), which lack most of the drug metabolism capability of hepatocytes. The role of unrecognized metabolites, therefore, may account in part for DILIsym's 20% prediction failure rate. The Initiative has begun to collect mitochondrial inhibition and oxidative stress data in culture systems containing primary human hepatocytes or a hepatoma cell line that maintains most of the metabolic capacity of human hepatocytes (HepaRG) (with and without addition of nonparenchymal cells). In 1 case involving a molecule that was not predicted to be hepatototoxic by the current DILIsym inputs (see **Fig. 2**), time-dependent appearance of oxidative stress was noted in cultures of primary human hepatocyte, likely reflecting a role for unrecognized metabolites (Merrie Mosedale, personal communication).

Mechanistic Insights

Several major insights regarding hepatoxicity mechanisms have evolved from the Initiative. These include importance of the mechanism underlying inhibition of bile acid transporters. When a drug is a competitive inhibitor of bile acid transporters, such as BSEP, as the hepatocyte concentration of the bile acids rises, the bile acids can out-compete the inhibitor to reduce the likelihood that toxic concentrations of bile acids in the hepatocyte will be achieved. In contrast, bile acids will be less able to override noncompetitive inhibition, and toxic concentrations are more likely to be achieved. The typically assessed concentration causing 50% inhibition of bile acid transport (IC50) does not identify mechanism of inhibition.

An example of where mechanism of inhibition of transporters was shown to be important in toxicity prediction involved an Amgen development program (Thousand Oaks, California). AMG 009 was a new drug candidate that demonstrated no liver safety signals in rat, dog, or monkey. Dose-dependent elevations in serum ALT, however, were observed in the phase 1 multiple dose-escalation clinical trial stopping clinical development. The program's backup drug, AMG 853, which also had clean preclinical toxicology studies, was advanced into clinical development and no liver safety signals were observed. Retrospective investigation revealed that both drugs were potent inhibitors of BSEP, which is the major transporter of bile acids into bile. When assessed by IC50, AMG 853 was a more potent inhibitor of BSEP than AMG 009. AMG 853 was determined, however, to be a competitive inhibitor of BSEP whereas AMG 009 was a noncompetitive inhibitor of BSEP. There was no indication that either drug caused oxidative stress or interfered with mitochondrial function. The PBPK predictions of hepatocyte drug concentration together with the mechanistic inhibition for BSEP, NTCP, and other efflux transporters of bile acids were determined and loaded into DILIsym and the outputs examined. For AMG 009, the predicted time-dependent and dose-dependent elevations in serum ALT were similar to those observed in the phase 1 trial (ie, without any manipulation to the model parameters) (**Fig. 4**). No ALT elevations greater than 3-times the ULN were predicted for AMG 853 (not shown), consistent with the clinical trial experience, and this was demonstrated to be largely due the fact that AMG 853 was a competitive inhibitor of BSEP. In addition, DILIsym modeling of both compounds in the rat version of DILIsym predicted no liver injury consistent with the preclinical findings. The difference between rat and human toxicity of AMG 009 could be largely related to the inherently less hepatotoxic profile of bile acids in the rat. This was the first example of importance of the mechanism of transporter inhibition in assessing the hepatotoxic potential of a new drug candidate, but there have since been others.[13]

The modeling also has provided novel insight into mechanisms underlying species differences in susceptibility to hepatotoxicity[16] and how structurally similar drug can have markedly different mechanisms of hepatotoxicity.[17] A more complete review of mechanistic insights that have evolved from the DILI-sim Initiative is available.[18]

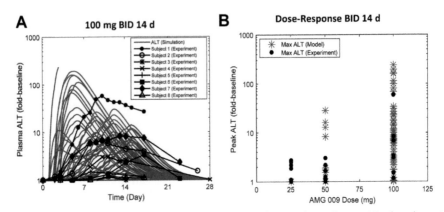

Fig. 4. Simulated serum ALT values (*red*) versus actual ALT values observed in the phase 1 clinical trials of AMG 009 (*black*) as a function of time on drug (*A*) and dose (*B*). Human_-mito_BA_v3A_6 Simpops were used for the simulations (17 NASH-like patients were excluded) and treatment stopped in the model when serum ALT exceeded 5-times the ULN.

The Prospective Use of DILIsym in Drug Development

When the model predicts a new drug candidate will cause serum ALT elevations, it is possible to vary the dosage to predict regimens that should minimize or eliminate ALT elevations. In addition, if elimination of ALT elevations is not achieved at doses predicted to be effective, the model can predict the frequency of liver chemistry monitoring and appropriate stopping criteria based on ALT value to avoid serious liver injury. The use of DILIsym in this way has been applied to several new drugs, including an antibiotic.[19]

An increasingly frequent application of DILIsym has been the assessment of the safety of next-in-class drugs when first-in-class drugs have had liver safety issues. This has been demonstrated retrospectively with drug pairs known to have discordant liver safety profiles. For example, DILIsym predicted the Parkinson treatment tolcapone to be hepatotoxic and that the next-in-class drug entacapone was safe.[20] Likewise, the model predicted troglitazone to be hepatotoxic and that the next-in-class drug pioglitazone was not.[21] The discordant liver safety of these drug pairs was already established; the use of the term, *prediction*, refers to the fact the model results were not fitted to the known safety profiles but were the results that were produced by the model without manipulation. A crucial test of the model is predictions made for new drug candidates before they enter clinical trials.[22] One such example involves 2 drugs to treat autosomal dominant polycystic kidney disease (ADPKD). The first-in-class drug, tolvaptan, was predicted by DILIsym to be potentially hepatotoxic in these patients whereas the next-in-class drug lixivaptan has been predicted by the model to be safe for the liver in the dosing proposed for this population.[23] Clinical trials of lixivaptan in ADPKD patients are under way. There currently are several other prospective clinical trials of next-in-class drugs, with the dosing regimens predicted by DILIsym to be safe.

Application of DILIsym to Improve Biomarker Interpretation

As discussed previously, DILIsym predicts the time-dependent death of hepatocytes and the subsequent release into circulation of biomarkers, typically ALT, and also the rise in serum bilirubin as an indicator of global liver dysfunction (see **Fig. 1**). Alternatively, if serial assessments of serum ALT are available in an actual patients experiencing hepatotoxicity, it is possible to fit the ALT kinetics to the model and, thereby, estimate the percent hepatocyte loss that the patient experienced. DILIsym actually creates a range of hepatocyte loss for a given ALT area under the curve, reflecting published variation in the content of ALT per hepatocyte and variation in the serum half-life of ALT. DILIsym was first used in this way to help interpret the significance of high peak serum ALT elevations (to 1000 IU/L) observed in healthy adults given a single injection of a toll-like receptor 5 agonist (a potential treatment of radiation sickness).[24] Although the peak serum ALT elevations observed exceeded 20-times the ULN, the serum ALT values peaked quickly and then fell at approximately the published half-life of the enzyme. This suggested a short duration of hepatocyte death, and this was confirmed by the DILIsym modeling. The peak hepatocyte fraction lost was estimated to be less than 5% in the most affected volunteer. In more prolonged liver injuries, it is important that regeneration of hepatocytes in response to hepatocyte loss is built into DILIsym, such that the functioning hepatocyte mass is predicted at any point during and after resolution of ongoing hepatocyte death. The modeling has shown that regeneration rate can be important in determining liver function, particularly during prolonged liver injuries.

An additional consideration is that the release of ALT per hepatocyte into blood is reduced during apoptosis versus necrosis and this is built into the model. By simply looking at the effect of switching mode of cell death in the model, it is possible to estimate the effect of the 2 cell death pathways on estimated hepatocyte loss. It also has been proposed that during a DILI event, the proportions of apoptosis versus necrosis can been estimated as the ratio of the caspase-cleaved fragment of cytokeratin 18 to the full-length K18, termed, *apoptotic index*, and this ratio is incorporated into DILIsym. The apoptotic index recently was used to estimate the peak loss of hepatocyte mass in healthy volunteers treated with alfa cimaglermin alfa,[25] a biologic agent proposed to treat congestive heart failure. In this case, the apoptotic index measured in archived serum samples supported apoptosis as the primary mode of liver cell death. The patient with the highest serum ALT peak value was predicted by DILIsym to have a peak reduction in hepatocyte mass of 12.5%. This was an important observation because this subject also experienced a rise in serum bilirubin exceeding 2-times the ULN (ie, a Hy's law case), prompting a clinical hold on the development program. According to DILIsym, the maximal 12.5% loss of hepatocytes was not sufficient to account for a rise in serum bilirubin. It was later shown that the rise in serum bilirubin may be explained by on-target effects of the drug independent of toxicity.[26] This modeling was presented as part of the regulatory communications aimed at removing the clinical hold on further development of this drug.

In addition to loss-of-function hepatocyte mass, DILIsym can predict elevations in direct and/or indirect bilirubin due to drug/metabolite inhibition of bilirubin transporters or inhibition of UGT1A1.[27] A more complete review of the use of DILIsym in biomarker interpretation is available.[24]

Future Applications of DILIsym

DILIsym has shown success in predicting dose-dependent hepatotoxicity, including species differences in susceptibility. A greater challenge is predicting the idiosyncratic DILI results now believed to frequently involve immune an attack on the liver.[28] Kupffer cell and recruited macrophage activation (the innate immune response in **Fig. 1**) are built into DILIsym.[29] Activation of innate immune responses in DILIsym not only promotes hepatocyte injury but also affects hepatocyte regeneration rates. It is now clear, however, that many cases of DILI result from an adaptive immune attack on the liver. Incorporation of adaptive immune responses in DILIsym has begun and is an area of emphasis going forward. This modeling should provide novel insights into mechanisms underlying idiosyncrasy as well as hepatotoxicity observed with immune modulators, such as the checkpoint inhibitors.[30]

Although adaptive immune responses are clearly important, the current versions of DILIsym successfully predicted the liver safety liability of 3 drugs that cause delayed idiosyncratic DILI, tolvaptan,[31] troglitazone,[21] and TAK-875.[13] This success supports the generally accepted concept that initiation of an adaptive immune attack requires drug-induced hepatocyte stress[28] and that this stress may in at least some cases be caused by the mechanisms already incorporated into DILIsym. Moreover, DILIsym predicted the several-month latency to peak serum ALT values observed in the clinical trials of troglitazone.[21] This may suggest that delayed presentation of idiosyncratic hepatotoxicity can occur without involving an adaptive immune response. Regardless of the role of adaptive immunity in DILI, according to current concepts, drug regimens predicted by DILIsym to not cause hepatotoxicity should have a reduced chance of causing idiosyncratic DILI.

Looking farther into the future, DILIsym modeling may be able to reduce the size of clinical trials needed to establish liver safety. Just like modeling of drug interactions based on ability of drugs to induce or inhibit drug-metabolizing enzymes is increasingly accepted in place of performing drug-drug interaction clinical trials, DILIsym modeling in simulated patient populations ultimately may be accepted by regulators in place of actual clinical safety trials. Finally, DILIsym may someday be useful to clinicians in managing liver safety risks in their patients. If DILIsym modeling has already been performed for a specific drug, it may be possible for a physician to access the model through a smartphone, input patient specific data such as underlying diseases (eg, NASH) or concomitant medications, and in return be given a quantitative assessment of risk of DILI at various dosing regimens for that patient. DILIsym also may be useful in identifying the culprit drug in a patient with DILI receiving multiple drugs that have been modeled in DILIsym.

SUMMARY

DILIsym has evolved from a successful ongoing public-private partnership. It has provided novel insight into mechanisms underlying DILI, including interpatient variation in susceptibility to DILI. It is increasingly used in decision making within industry, and DILIsym modeling results are increasingly included in regulatory communications. It seems likely that DILIsym and QST efforts focused on other organs will improve the safety of new drugs while improving the efficiency of drug development.

REFERENCES

1. Bloomingdale P, Housand C, Apgar JF, et al. Quantitative systems toxicology. Curr Opin Toxicol 2017;4:79–87.

2. Howell BA, Siler SQ, Barton HA, et al. Development of quantitative systems pharmacology and toxicology models within consortia: experiences and lessons learned through DILIsym development. Drug Discov Today Dis Models 2016; 22(Supplement C):5–13.

3. Howell BA, Yang Y, Kumar R, et al. In vitro to in vivo extrapolation and species response comparisons for drug-induced liver injury (DILI) using DILIsym™: a mechanistic, mathematical model of DILI. J Pharmacokinet Pharmacodyn 2012; 39(5):527–41.

4. Shoda LKM, Woodhead JL, Siler SQ, et al. Linking physiology to toxicity using DILIsym®, a mechanistic mathematical model of drug-induced liver injury. Biopharm Drug Dispos 2014;35(1):33–49.

5. Woodhead JL, Howell BA, Yang Y, et al. An analysis of N-acetylcysteine treatment for acetaminophen overdose using a systems model of drug-induced liver injury. Pharmacol Exp Ther 2012;342(2):529–40.

6. Howell BA, Siler SQ, Watkins PB. Use of a systems model of drug-induced liver injury (DILIsym®) to elucidate the mechanistic differences between acetaminophen and its less-toxic isomer, AMAP, in mice. Toxicol Lett 2014;226(2):163–72.

7. Guo C, Yang K, Brouwer KR, et al. Prediction of altered bile acid disposition due to inhibition of multiple transporters: an integrated approach using sandwich-cultured hepatocytes, mechanistic modeling, and simulation. Pharmacol Exp Ther 2016;358(2):324–33.

8. He K, Cai L, Shi Q, et al. Inhibition of MDR3 activity in human hepatocytes by drugs associated with liver injury. Chem Res Toxicol 2015;28(10):1987–90.

9. Portmann B, Talbot IC, Day DW, et al. Histopathological changes in the liver following a paracetamol overdose: correlation with clinical and biochemical parameters. Pathol 1975;117(3):169–81.

10. Church RJ, Watkins PB. The transformation in biomarker detection and management of drug-induced liver injury. Liver Int 2017;37(11):1582–90.

11. Perez-Carreras M, Del Hoyo P, Martin MA, et al. Defective hepatic mitochondrial respiratory chain in patients with nonalcoholic steatohepatitis. Hepatology 2003;38(4):999–1007.

12. Watkins PB, Desai M, Berkowitz SD, et al. Evaluation of drug-induced serious hepatotoxicity (eDISH): application of this data organization approach to phase III clinical trials of rivaroxaban after total hip or knee replacement surgery. Drug Saf 2011;34(3):243–52.

13. Longo DM, Woodhead JL, Walker P, et al. Quantitative systems toxicology analysis of in vitro mechanistic assays reveals importance of bile acid accumulation and mitochondrial dysfunction in TAK-875-induced liver injury. Toxicol Sci 2019;167(2):458–67.

14. Park BK, Kitteringham NR, Maggs JL, et al. The role of metabolic activation in drug-induced hepatotoxicity. Annu Rev Pharmacol Toxicol 2005;45:177–202.

15. Iorga A, Dara L, Kaplowitz N. Drug-induced liver injury: cascade of events leading to cell death, apoptosis or necrosis. Int J Mol Sci 2017;18(5) [pii:E1018].

16. Battista C, Yang K, Stahl SH, et al. Using quantitative systems toxicology to investigate observed species differences in CKA-mediated hepatotoxicity. Toxicol Sci 2018;166(1):123–30.

17. Woodhead JL, Yang K, Oldach D, et al. Analyzing the mechanisms behind macrolide antibiotic-induced liver injury using quantitative systems toxicology modeling. Pharm Res 2019;36(3):48.

18. Watkins PB. The DILI-sim initiative: insights into hepatotoxicity mechanisms and biomarker interpretation. Clin Transl Sci 2019;12(2):122–9.

19. Woodhead JL, Paech F, Maurer M, et al. Prediction of safety margin and optimization of dosing protocol for a novel antibiotic using quantitative systems pharmacology modeling. Clin Transl Sci 2018;11(5):498–505.

20. Longo DM, Yang Y, Watkins PB, et al. Elucidating differences in the hepatotoxic potential of tolcapone and entacapone with DILIsym®, a mechanistic model of drug-induced liver injury. CPT Pharmacometrics Syst Pharmacol 2016;5(1):31–9.

21. Yang K, Woodhead JL, Watkins PB, et al. Systems pharmacology modeling predicts delayed presentation and species differences in bile Acid-mediated troglitazone hepatotoxicity. Clin Pharmacol Ther 2014;96(5):589–98.

22. Shon J, Abernethy DR. Application of systems pharmacology to explore mechanisms of hepatotoxicity. Clin Pharmacol Ther 2014;96(5):536–7.

23. Howell BA, Woodhead JL, Pellegrini L, et al. Liver safety comparison of two treatments for autosomal-dominant polycystic Kidney disease (ADPKD) using quantitative systems toxicology software (DILIsym). Baltimore (MD): American Association of Pharmceutical Scientists; 2018.

24. Church RJ, Watkins PB. In silico modeling to optimize interpretation of liver safety biomarkers in clinical trials. Exp Biol Med (Maywood) 2018;243(3):300–7.

25. Longo DM, Generaux GT, Howell BA, et al. Refining liver safety risk assessment: application of mechanistic modeling and serum biomarkers to cimaglermin alfa (GGF2) clinical trials. Clin Pharmacol Ther 2017;102(6):961–9.

26. Mosedale M, Button D, Jackson JP, et al. Transient changes in hepatic physiology that alter bilirubin and bile acid transport may explain elevations in liver chemistries observed in clinical trials of GGF2 (cimaglermin alfa). Toxicol Sci 2018; 161(2):401–11.

27. Yang K, Battista C, Woodhead JL, et al. Systems pharmacology modeling of drug-induced hyperbilirubinemia: differentiating hepatotoxicity and inhibition of enzymes/transporters. Clin Pharmacol Ther 2017;101(4):501–9.

28. Mosedale M, Watkins PB. Drug-induced liver injury: advances in mechanistic understanding that will inform risk management. Invited "state-of-the-art" review. Clin Pharmacol Ther 2017;101(4):469–80.

29. Shoda LK, Battista C, Siler SQ, et al. Mechanistic modelling of drug-induced liver injury: investigating the role of innate immune responses. Gene Regul Syst Bio 2017;11. 1177625017696074.

30. Suzman DL, Pelosof L, Rosenberg A, et al. Hepatotoxicity of immune checkpoint inhibitors: an evolving picture of risk associated with a vital class of immunotherapy agents. Liver Int 2018;38(6):976–87.

31. Woodhead JL, Brock WJ, Roth SE, et al. Application of a mechanistic model to evaluate putative mechanisms of tolvaptan drug-induced liver injury and identify patient susceptibility factors. Toxicol Sci 2017;155(1):61–74.

Liver Histology
Diagnostic and Prognostic Features

Billel Gasmi, MD[a], David E. Kleiner, MD, PhD[b],*

KEYWORDS

- Hepatotoxicity • Acute hepatitis • Cholestatic hepatitis • Hepatic necrosis
- Nodular regenerative hyperplasia

KEY POINTS

- Liver biopsy can provide useful information on differential diagnosis and severity of injury in drug-induced liver injury.
- Hepatic pathologists are expert consultants able to interpret histologic findings in light of complex clinical information.
- The pathologist defines the hepatic pattern of injury, which is closely related to the histologic differential diagnosis.
- A liver biopsy may be the only way to diagnose certain injury types, in particular, vascular injury.
- The severity and character of the histologic injury may relate to prognosis.

Drug-induced liver injury (DILI) is one of the most challenging aspects of hepatic pathology both because of its inherent complexity and because a patient's comorbidities may interfere with interpretation. Biopsies may be performed for several reasons. Usually, a liver biopsy is done in suspected DILI to aid in diagnosis because of some clinical uncertainty. A biopsy also may be used to assess the severity of the liver damage or to exclude serious findings like duct loss, necrosis, or advanced fibrosis. Frequently there are issues of differential diagnosis. There may be a known preexisting liver disease or a patient's comorbidities may have complex secondary effects on the liver. With newer drugs that have little or no record of liver injury, a biopsy may provide

Disclosure Statement: The authors have nothing to disclose. Dr D.E. Kleiner and Dr B. Gasmi shared responsibility for preparing and critical review of the article, including all figures and tables.
Funding Acknowledgment: This review was supported by the Intramural Research Program of the NIH, National Cancer Institute.
[a] Laboratory of Pathology, National Cancer Institute, 10 Center Drive, Building 10, Room 2S235, MSC1500, Bethesda, MD 20892, USA; [b] Post-Mortem Section, Laboratory of Pathology, National Cancer Institute, 10 Center Drive, Building 10, Room 2S235, MSC1500, Bethesda, MD 20892, USA
* Corresponding author.
E-mail address: kleinerd@mail.nih.gov

information on the mechanism of injury. This was the case with the experimental agent fialuridine, where liver tissue from biopsy and explant provided the confirmation that mitochondrial injury was the source of the problem.[1,2]

The role of the pathologist in evaluating cases of DILI is to provide expert interpretation of the tissue changes considering a patient's medical and pharmaceutical history. Because of the potential complexity of these cases, a systematic approach is recommended (**Box 1**). The first step is objective and unbiased evaluation of the changes, organizing them into the defined patterns of injury common to many liver diseases. **Table 1** and the body of this review highlight the most common patterns of significant injury that have been identified in cases of DILI.[3,4] Tumors are excluded from the classification, because the evaluation in such cases is focused on tumor diagnosis rather than attributing the tumor development to a particular agent. Once the pattern(s) of injury are defined, the pathologist must correlate the findings with the history, sorting out findings that can be attributed to nondrug etiologies, which may require workup for unusual causes of liver injury. Resources are available for finding patterns of histologic injury due to drugs. These include the National Intitutes of Health LiverTox Web site (https://livertox.nih.gov/) and DILI book chapters in references devoted to hepatic pathology. Drugs that have been recently approved (especially checkpoint inhibitors,[5] tyrosine kinase inhibitors,[6] monoclonal antibodies,[7] and small molecule immunomodulators[8]) may require searches of the biomedical literature databases. The final pathology report should include information on the pattern of injury, the severity of injury, and the differential diagnosis.

NECROINFLAMMATORY PATTERNS

Histologic injury in DILI often manifests as inflammation or hepatocellular necrosis or a combination of the 2 (**Fig. 1**). More than a third of cases of suspected DILI in the DILI Network (DILIN) show significant necroinflammatory injury without visible cholestasis, and, if cases of acute hepatitis with mild cholestasis are included, the total reaches nearly half.[3] There are 2 basic patterns of inflammation, which the authors have termed, *acute hepatitis* and *chronic hepatitis*, although it should be remembered that these represent histologic patterns important for differential diagnosis and do not necessarily convey information about the time course of the injury. Both patterns can range in severity from mild to marked and distinction between the 2 can be difficult at both extremes.

Acute hepatitic patterns involve the parenchyma more than the portal areas, with hepatocyte apoptosis and numerous foci of lymphocytes and macrophages

---

Box 1
Systematic approach to the histologic evaluation of potential drug-induced liver injury

1. Identify the pattern of injury

2. Identify the suspect agents
   a. Drug, herbal, environmental exposures
   b. Appropriate time line?
   c. Appropriate histologic injury pattern?

3. Exclude other causes of injury (or not)

4. Draw conclusions
   a. Comment on the elements in step 2
   b. Comment on any potential alternative etiologies that may require additional testing

Table 1
Non-neoplastic patterns of injury observed in drug-induced liver injury and their differential diagnosis

	Pattern	Characteristic Features	Common Alternate Etiologies	Uncommon Alternate Etiologies
Necroinflammatory	Acute (lobular) hepatitis	Predominantly lobular inflammation with/without confluent or bridging necrosis; lobular disarray; absence of or only minimal cholestasis	Acute viral or autoimmune hepatitis	
	Chronic (portal) hepatitis	Portal inflammation with interface hepatitis, with or without portal-based fibrosis; no cholestasis	Chronic viral or autoimmune diseases	Early PBC/PSC, EBV, or CMV-associated hepatitis (mononucleosis pattern), collagen-vascular disease, celiac disease, CVID
	Granulomatous hepatitis	Typically non-necrotizing granulomatous inflammation dominates pattern	Sarcoidosis, PBC	Fungal, mycobacterial, and atypical bacterial or rickettsial infections, CVID
	Massive or submassive necrosis	Complete loss of hepatocytes over large areas, with regenerative nodules	Fulminant viral hepatitis	
	Zonal coagulative necrosis	Zone 3 or 1 coagulative necrosis, usually without significant inflammation	Hypoxic-ischemic injury (zone 3)	Necrotizing viral infections (usually nonzonal)
Cholestatic	Cholestatic hepatitis	Acute or chronic hepatitis pattern plus zone 3 cholestasis	Acute viral or autoimmune hepatitis	Progressive familial intrahepatic cholestasis
	Acute intrahepatic cholestasis	Hepatocellular and/or canalicular cholestasis in zone 3, minimal inflammation	Sepsis, acute large duct obstruction, postsurgical jaundice	Benign recurrent intrahepatic cholestasis
	Chronic cholestasis (vanishing bile duct syndrome)	Duct sclerosis and loss, periportal cholestasis, portal-based fibrosis, copper accumulation	PSC	Biliary tree infections in the immunosuppressed patient, ductopenic GVHD, idiopathic adulthood ductopenia, Langerhans cell histiocytosis, IgG4-related systemic sclerosis
	Chronic cholestasis (PBC-like cholangiodestructive)	Florid duct injury with duct loss, periportal cholestasis, copper	Primary biliary cirrhosis, autoimmune cholangitis, chronic large duct obstruction	Progressive familial intrahepatic cholestasis

(continued on next page)

Table 1
(continued)

	Pattern	Characteristic Features	Common Alternate Etiologies	Uncommon Alternate Etiologies
Steatotic	Microvesicular steatosis	Diffuse microvesicular steatosis	Alcohol, fatty liver of pregnancy	
	Macrovesicular steatosis	Macrovesicular steatosis without significant portal or lobular inflammation, no cholestasis	Very common finding in general population, alcohol, obesity, diabetes	Celiac disease
	Steatohepatitis	Zone 3 ballooning injury, sinusoidal fibrosis, Mallory bodies, variable inflammation, and steatosis	As for macrovesicular steatosis	
Vascular	Sinusoidal dilation/peliosis	Sinusoidal alterations, may have sinusoidal fibrosis	Artifactual, acute congestion, nearby mass lesions	Bacillary angiomatosis
	VOD/SOS/Budd-Chiari	Occlusion or loss of central veins, thrombosis, with or without central hemorrhage and necrosis		
	Hepatoportal sclerosis	Disappearance of portal veins		
	Nodular regenerative hyperplasia	Diffuse nodular transformation, may have sinusoidal fibrosis	Collagen-vascular diseases, lymphoproliferative diseases	Arteriohepatic dysplasia
Miscellaneous changes and pigment accumulations	Glycogenosis	Diffuse hepatocyte swelling with very pale bluish-gray cytoplasm	Type 1 diabetes mellitus, obesity	
	Ground-glass change	Diffuse homogenization of cell cytoplasm due to induction of smooth endoplasmic reticulum		
	Cytoplasmic inclusions	Discrete PAS-positive or -negative cytoplasmic inclusions	α_1-Antitrypsin deficiency, long-standing hepatic congestion, megamitochondria	
	Gold pigment	Granular black pigment in Kupffer cells	Anthracosis	Malarial pigment

Abbreviations: CMV, cytomegalovirus; CVID, common variable immune deficiency; EBV, epstein-barr virus; GVHD, graft versus host disease; IgG, immunoglobulin G; PSC, primary sclerosing cholangitis.

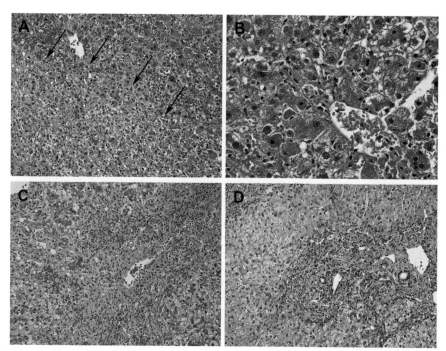

Fig. 1. Necroinflammatory patterns. (*A, B*) Acute hepatitis due to azithromycin. There were irregular, nonzonal regions of necrosis (*arrows* [*A*]) whereas numerous apoptotic hepatocytes and foci of lobular inflammation were seen near central veins (*B*). (*C*) Zone 3 necrosis due to acetaminophen. A mild mononuclear infiltrate is present in the necrotic zone. (*D*) Chronic hepatitis-like portal inflammation due to atorvastatin. (*A*) Hematoxylin-Eosin, original magnification ×200; (*B*) Hematoxylin-Eosin, original magnification ×400; (*C*) Hematoxylin-Eosin, original magnification ×100; and (*D*) Hematoxylin-Eosin, original magnification ×200.

disrupting the normal sinusoidal architecture of the liver, a finding termed *lobular disarray*. Lobular disarray often is associated with features of regeneration, including mitotic activity and hepatocyte rosettes. Portal inflammation with interface hepatitis also may be severe but in proportion to the parenchymal injury. Plasma cells and eosinophils may be seen, particularly in portal areas. Plasma cells at the periphery of the portal area raise a differential diagnosis of autoimmune hepatitis. There may be perivenular (zone 3) necrosis. This latter finding has been associated with particular agents, including diclofenac[9] and ipilimumab.[10] When cholestasis is present in severe acute hepatitis, it usually is mild and difficult to identify. Such cases are classified as acute cholestatic hepatitis or acute hepatitis with cholestasis. In studies, they may be grouped with either acute hepatitis without evident cholestasis or as one of the forms of cholestatic hepatitis.[3] Many drugs can show an acute hepatitic pattern, including checkpoint inhibitors,[11] infliximab (and other tumor necrosis factor α antagonists),[12] isoniazid, nonsteroidal anti-inflammatory agents, and agents used to treat psychiatric disorders. Severe cases of acute hepatitis present with aminotransferases elevated 10-fold to 30-fold above the upper limit of normal and usually are jaundiced.[3]

Chronic (or portal-predominant) hepatitic patterns resemble chronic viral hepatitis histologically, with portal inflammation visible at low magnification and only mild to moderate parenchymal inflammation. Hepatocyte rosettes can be seen when the overall inflammation is severe, but the presence of lobular disarray prompts classification as an acute hepatitic pattern. Similarly, cholestasis is not seen in this pattern of injury—these cases should be considered a form of cholestatic hepatitis. Fibrosis sometimes is present and may bridge between portal areas as in the case of nitrofurantoin injury.[13] Many of the drugs that cause acute hepatitis also may show a chronic hepatitic pattern, such as nitrofurantoin,[14] minocycline,[14] isoniazid,[15] and atorvastatin.[16] Clinically, patients with chronic hepatitis pattern present with only modest elevation in aminotransferases and normal bilirubin levels.

Hepatocellular necrosis is a frequent finding in DILI. In the DILIN study, a quarter of the biopsies showed some degree of confluent necrosis, and most of the time it followed a zone 3–centered distribution.[3] When necrosis is severe, it may involve multiple contiguous hepatic acini and clinically these patients present with fulminant hepatic failure. Zone 1 necrosis is rare and usually related to a direct hepatic toxin like phosphorus rather than a drug.[17] Zone 3 coagulative necrosis is the classic injury pattern of acetaminophen and it is related to the accumulation of the toxic metabolite in a susceptible population of cells. There is minimal inflammation with acetaminophen, with infiltration of macrophages and some neutrophils into the region of necrosis (see **Fig. 1**C). Pure zone 3 necrosis without significant inflammation is unusual in other drugs and should prompt a search for occlusive vascular injury.

Other patterns of necroinflammatory injury include granulomatous hepatitis and the sinusoidal lymphocytosis pattern. The latter is the typical inflammatory pattern for EBV-related hepatitis but also may be seen with some drugs, such as phenytoin.[18] This pattern is most similar to the chronic hepatitic pattern because there is portal inflammation with less lobular inflammation. In sinusoidal lymphocytosis, there is beading of lymphocytes and macrophages in the sinuses without infiltration into the cords of liver cells. In situ hybridization for EBV should be performed to exclude that diagnosis. Granulomatous hepatitis is diagnosed when granulomatous inflammation is dominant. Microgranulomas, which are small collections of macrophages in the range of 1 to 3 hepatocytes in size are frequently observed in DILI and in non-DILI liver disease and should not be used to classify the case as granulomatous hepatitis. The granulomas in DILI-related granulomatous hepatitis are larger and do not have necrotic centers (which would suggest infection). They may be well formed and sarcoid-like, as has been seen with interferon, or poorly formed, with infiltration by lymphocytes and ill-defined edges. Fibrin ring granulomas, an unusual type of lipogranuloma centered around a lipid vacuole and surrounded by fibrin and epithelioid histiocytes, have been observed in several types of DILI, including injury due to allopurinol[19] and checkpoint inhibitors.[20] Fungal and mycobacterial infection need to be excluded, particularly in immunosuppressed patients. Depending on the location of the granulomas, other diseases, such as primary biliary cholangitis (PBC), may need to be considered.

Finally, the inflammatory infiltrate may be mild, in the range of reactive forms of hepatitis observed in collagen-vascular diseases. Such cases might have a sprinkling of inflammation in the portal areas with an occasional focus of interface hepatitis and widely scattered foci of lobular inflammation. The presence of clusters of pigmented macrophages may suggest a more severe hepatitis has come and gone, but there may be little to suggest any injury. The clinical significance of these mild forms of injury is unknown.

CHOLESTATIC INJURY PATTERNS

Cholestasis may be observed in 2 basic forms in the liver: as the accumulation of bile or as the accumulation of bile salts. In the former situation, bile can be found within hepatocytes, dilated canaliculi, cholangioles or the interlobular ducts. Bile pigment also can be found in macrophages, particularly in zone 3. Cytoplasmic bile, whether in macrophages or hepatocytes, can be difficult to differentiate from other pigments, such as hemosiderin and lipofuscin. Special stains may be useful in differentiating pigments. Bile stains can be used to demonstrate bile directly, and iron and copper have a pale counterstain that allows the natural greenish-brown bile pigment to be more clearly seen. Bile within canaliculi and duct structures can be identified without the use of special stains. The location of the bile is important because ductal and ductular bile accumulation are unusual in DILI. Bile salts accumulate in the periportal hepatocytes in chronic cholestasis, causing the cytoplasm to become pale and vacuolated. This change may be termed *cholate stasis*, *pseudoxanthomatous change*, or *feathery degeneration*, depending on the age of the publication. Copper accumulates in these hepatocytes and can be identified directly with copper stains or indirectly with orcein or Victoria blue stains. Immunohistochemistry for keratin 7 may be positive in periportal hepatocytes in chronic cholestasis.

There are 3 main patterns of cholestatic liver injury seen in DILI (**Fig. 2**), although it is possible to subdivide these into additional categories based on the non-DILI differential diagnosis. The most common pattern is the mixed pattern of cholestatic hepatitis, accounting for almost 30% of the cases in the DILIN study.[3] These cases have portal and/or parenchymal inflammation as well as canalicular and hepatocellular

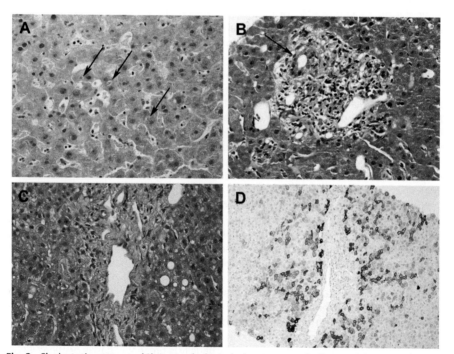

Fig. 2. Cholestatic patterns. (*A*) Acute cholestasis due to an anabolic steroid. Canalicular bile plugs in zone 3 (*arrows*) are present but there is minimal inflammation. (*B*) Bile duct injury (*arrow*) due to amoxicillin-clavulanate. Cholestasis (not pictured) was seen in zone 3. (*C, D*) Chronic cholestasis and bile duct loss due to gabapentin. The portal areas show no ducts, as confirmed by staining for keratin 7 (*D*). (*A*) Hematoxylin-Eosin, original magnification ×400; (*B*) Hematoxylin-Eosin, original magnification ×400; (*C*) Hematoxylin-Eosin, original magnification ×400; and (*D*) Keratin 7 immunohistochemistery, original magification ×200).

cholestasis. The cholestasis begins in zone 3 but can be extensive. The distribution and severity of inflammation can replicate the inflammatory patterns, outlined previously. Cases of acute hepatitic inflammatory injury usually have mild cholestasis that may be difficult to identify without special stains. When the hepatitic component is less severe, the cholestasis is usually easier to identify. Other features of cholestatic injury, including bile duct injury or loss and hepatocellular swelling from cytoplasmic bile, also may be present. Liver enzymes show a bimodal distribution. The cases of acute hepatitis with cholestasis present clinically like acute hepatitis, with marked elevations in aminotransferases and jaundice. In contrast, cases of inflammation and more cholestasis have ratios of aminotransferases and alkaline phosphatase in the cholestatic range.[3] Cholestatic hepatitis has a non-DILI differential diagnosis that varies according the inflammatory pattern.

When the inflammatory component disappears but the cholestasis remains, the pattern becomes acute or intrahepatic cholestasis. This is the classic pattern of injury of the contraceptive and anabolic steroids[21] but may be seen with other drugs as well. There may be a minimal inflammatory infiltrate: scattered lymphocytes in portal areas and clusters of pigmented macrophages in zone 3. As with cholestatic hepatitis, duct injury or loss may be seen. Duct loss without other chronic cholestatic features may occur as in cases of azithromycin DILI.[22]

Cases of features of chronic cholestasis tend to show increased fibrosis associated with ductular reaction. The bile ducts usually show some degree of injury, which may mimic the duct injury of PBC or primary sclerosing cholangitis, but duct loss is not required. This pattern of injury is important to recognize because it may take longer for the liver enzymes to return to normal compared with other types of liver injury.[23,24]

STEATOSIS AND STEATOHEPATITIS

Liver diseases related to macrovesicular steatosis, which include both alcoholic liver disease and nonalcoholic fatty liver disease (NAFLD), are among the most common in the world. When these patterns of injury are present in a suspected case of DILI, it is necessary to show that the common etiologies of fatty liver disease are not responsible for the changes. Some agents, such as tamoxifen[25] or methotrexate,[26] can mimic the patterns of NAFLD exactly. This includes mimicking steatohepatitis, with zone 3 ballooning injury and perisinusoidal fibrosis (**Fig. 3**). Careful attention to other changes, such as cholestasis, marked degrees of inflammation, vascular injury, and numerous apoptotic hepatocytes, may be necessary to identify features that might indicate the presence of drug injury. Demonstration that drug injury was present may require follow-up after discontinuation of the suspect drug and resolution, as was the result in a case of tamoxifen injury highlighted by the DILIN investigators in their study of chronic liver injury.[23]

Some drugs interfere with lipid metabolism or induce steatogenic states by altering peripheral insulin resistance and this fact may provide an explanation for hepatic steatosis. This is particularly true for drugs that cause mitochondrial injury. Acetaminophen can interfere with mitochondrial function in several ways[27] and steatosis often is seen in acetaminophen injury. Mitochondrial injury usually is present in cases of microvesicular steatosis. Microvesicular steatosis is defined as a foamy change in the hepatocyte cytoplasm with innumerable tiny vacuoles that fill the cytoplasm. Diffuse microvesicular change throughout the biopsy defines the pattern of microvesicular steatosis. There is limited differential diagnosis for diffuse microvesicular steatosis and almost all of the causes are drugs or toxins. Notable drugs associated with microvesicular steatosis include salicylates,[28] amiodarone,[29] linezolid[30] and valproic acid.[31] The

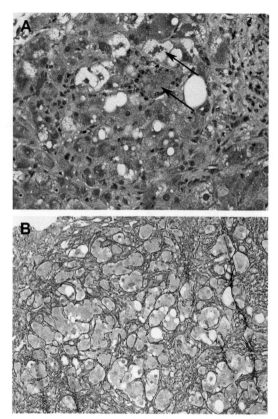

Fig. 3. Steatohepatitis due to methotrexate. (*A*) Ballooning injury with Mallory-Denk bodies (*arrows*). (*B*) Extensive perisinusoidal fibrosis seen in a reticulin stain. (*A*) Hematoxylin-Eosin, original magnification ×400 and (*B*) Reticulin, original magnification ×200.

nondrug causes include environmental toxins, alcohol (acute foamy degeneration), and fatty liver of pregnancy.

VASCULAR INJURY

Most of the DILI literature focuses on the hepatocyte, which is the most common target. Hepatocyte function and survival also can be secondarily affected by vascular injury. Drug-induced vascular injury can occur at any level, from the small portal veins to the large hepatic veins. Starting from the outflow side, oral contraceptives and other drugs that interfere with coagulation can cause hepatic venous thrombosis. Affected segments of the liver show massive hemorrhage and necrosis. Thrombi may be seen in the larger veins. Veno-occlusive disease/sinusoidal obstruction syndrome (VOD/SOS) occurs with injury to the endothelium of the sinusoids and small hepatic veins. Mainly associated with stem cell transplant preparative regimens, VOD/SOS is diagnosed by characteristic narrowing and occlusion of hepatic veins by cells and loose connective tissue (**Fig. 4D**). The sinusoidal injury, although present, is difficult to recognize histologically, particularly when there is secondary hemorrhage and necrosis of perivenular hepatocytes. Venular endotheliitis with hemorrhage but without venous occlusion

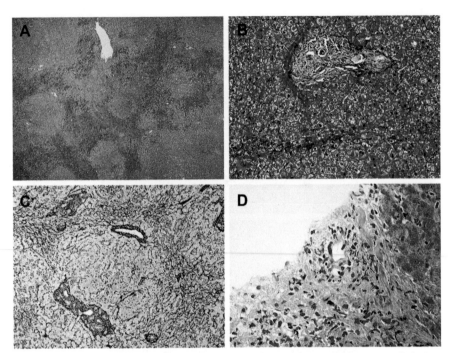

Fig. 4. Vascular injury patterns. (*A–C*) NRH and hepatoportal sclerosis due to oxaliplatin. A low-magnification overview shows areas of vascular congestion outlining nodules (A). The Masson trichrome stain showed that most of the small portal areas lacked a vein (*B*). Reticulin staining shows the characteristic nodular regeneration (*C*). (*D*) Veno-occlusive changes after hematopoietic stem cell transplantation. A small vein shows nearly complete occlusion by loose collagen and cells. (*A*) Hematoxylin-Eosin, original magnification ×40; (*B*) Masson trichrome, original magnification ×200; (*C*) Reticulin, original magnification ×100; (*D*) Masson trichrome, original magnification ×400.

may be a component of acute hepatitis and has been reported as a finding in checkpoint inhibitor injury.[11] As a finding in cases of suspected DILI in the DILIN study, venous endotheliitis was more common than either portal vein injury or VOD/SOS.[3]

Injury to the sinuses and portal veins may be insidious, unlike the more dramatic clinical presentations stemming from outflow obstruction. Oxaliplatin[32] and the purine analogues[33] have been associated with nodular regenerative hyperplasia (NRH) and noncirrhotic portal hypertension (**Fig. 4**). NRH may be easily overlooked on needle biopsies if reticulin stains are not performed or the pathologist is not comfortable with interpreting the changes. The mercaptopurines also may cause a cholestatic hepatitis, which may obscure underlying NRH. The key feature to identify is regular variation in hepatocyte plate width, with areas of compressed, atrophic liver cell plates arcing around zones of widened liver cell plates. Portal vein injury (hepatoportal sclerosis) is another subtle injury that has been observed with oxaliplatin and other agents. The portal veins may be slit-like or disappear or herniate into adjacent sinusoids. Because these changes may be seen on occasion in normal liver, it is important to assess each portal area to make sure that the findings are consistent throughout the biopsy. Sinusoidal dilation may accompany both NRH and portal venopathy.

BIOPSIES WITH MINIMAL CHANGES

Sometimes the liver biopsy shows minimal changes or even look normal. As discussed previously, injury to the portal veins and NRH can be subtle but should be excluded on any biopsy with an apparently unremarkable appearance on routine stains, particularly if there is any suggestion of portal hypertension in the history. Patients who have recovered from a mild acute hepatitic injury may show only clusters of pigmented, periodic acid–Schiff (PAS)-positive macrophages in the parenchyma, marking the location of hepatocyte loss (**Fig. 5**). Other subtle changes include hepatocyte cytoplasmic inclusions or alterations. Ground-glass–like inclusions that mimic those of hepatitis B may be seen associated with polypharmacy in immunosuppressed patients. These often are strongly positive with PAS and variably sensitive to diastase digestion. Diffuse ground-glass–like changes may be seen with activation of endoplasmic reticulum or with diffuse glycogenosis. Czeczok and colleagues[34] have outlined the entities associated with near-normal liver biopsies and it may be helpful to use these entities as a checklist when evaluating such cases.

PROGNOSTIC INFORMATION

Commonly used serum markers of liver injury (aminotransferases and alkaline phosphatase) are not able to reliably predict clinical outcomes of DILI. Although there is a great interest in identifying novel serum and genetic biomarkers for DILI diagnosis and prognosis, current prediction algorithms, such as Acute Liver Failure Study Group (ALFSG) index,[35] combine clinical and laboratory values but do not include histologic findings.

Liver histology can provide prognostic information assisting clinical management. In the DILIN study,[3] necrosis, fibrosis, microvesicular steatosis, cholangiolar cholestasis, ductular reaction, neutrophils, and portal venopathy were all associated with severe outcom, whereas granulomas and eosinophils[3,36] were more likely to be noted in milder cases. In other studies, the degree of necrosis and the presence of ductular reaction were also found critical in predicting survival. Liver biopsy with more than 75% necrosis was associated with significant transplant-free mortality in a patient population with fulminant liver failure due to autoimmune hepatitis, DILI, or hepatitis virus infection.[37]

Liver biopsy also may raise concerns for delayed recovery from DILI. Biochemically cholestatic injury has been associated with persistent liver enzyme abnormalities.[23]

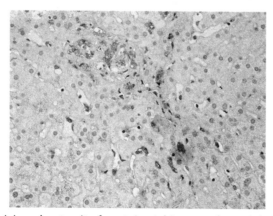

Fig. 5. Resolving injury due to nitrofurantoin. A biopsy performed during the resolving phase of DILI shows minimal changes, seen as clusters of pigmented macrophages highlighted by a PAS stain with diastase digestion (Periodic acid-Schiff with diastase, original magnification ×400).

When cases were investigated with liver biopsy, it was shown that patients with bile duct loss were more likely to develop chronic liver injury. Bile duct loss during acute cholestatic hepatitis was found to be an early indicator of possible vanishing bile duct syndrome.[38]

Histologic findings can also guide the identification of serologic prognostic markers. After necrosis and apoptosis were shown to be associated with a worsened laboratory versus clinical course in animal models,[39] a serum-based apoptotic index was proposed as as a prognostic tool.[35,39] The index estimates the degree of apoptosis and necrosis in liver injury by measuring the ratio of full-length cytokeratin 18 and caspase-cleaved cytokeratin 18.

PRACTICAL CONSIDERATIONS

There have been no systematic studies on the utility of liver biopsy in the diagnosis or management of DILI, although suspected DILI is a reasonable indication for liver biopsy.[40] The European Association for the Study of the Liver clinical practice guidelines[41] for DILI recommend a liver biopsy in patients suspected of having DILI when serology raises the possibility of autoimmune hepatitis, if suspected DILI progresses, or if DILI fails to resolve on withdrawal of the causal agent. More broadly, a liver biopsy may be considered during the investigation of selected patients suspected of suffering from DILI, because liver histology can provide information supporting the diagnosis of DILI or an alternative. As discussed previously, the pattern of liver biopsy may provide diagnostic information by matching known patterns of DILI or by identifying alternative explanations for the injury. The liver biopsy may identify potential etiologies that require additional clinical work-up to exclude. The character and severity of the injury (necrosis, inflammation, and duct loss) may be useful in patient management on a case-by-case basis. Adequacy of the liver biopsy is important, particularly when evaluating bile duct and portal veins. Existing guidelines for adequacy are based on large studies of chronic liver diseases, which have a consistent pattern of injury. In cases of DILI, the condition of the liver is unknown, so the minimum biopsy size should err on the large side: at least 3 cm of tissue core taken with a large needle size (16 gauge).[40]

SUMMARY

Liver biopsy can be a useful tool in the diagnosis of DILI, particularly in more complex clinical situations or when underlying liver disease is present. Pathologists should carefully evaluate the biopsy to establish the pattern and severity of injury and then correlate these observations with the patient's history, laboratory tests, and imaging findings. Direct communication with the clinical team can be helpful to clarify the findings and to discuss possible additional clinical evaluation. The final pathology report should include the pathologic findings and clinical-pathologic correlation. The pathologic diagnosis or report discussion should include a comment on the likelihood of a specific drug cause based on the histologic examination. This approach will ensure that the information from the liver biopsy is used to maximum clinical benefit.

REFERENCES

1. Kleiner DE, Gaffey MJ, Sallie R, et al. Histopathologic changes associated with fialuridine hepatotoxicity. Mod Pathol 1997;10(3):192–9.
2. McKenzie R, Fried MW, Sallie R, et al. Hepatic failure and lactic acidosis due to fialuridine (FIAU), an investigational nucleoside analogue for chronic hepatitis B. N Engl J Med 1995;333(17):1099–105.

3. Kleiner DE, Chalasani NP, Lee WM, et al. Hepatic histological findings in suspected drug-induced liver injury: systematic evaluation and clinical associations. Hepatology 2014;59(2):661–70.
4. Popper H, Rubin E, Cardiol D, et al. Drug-induced liver disease: a penalty for progress. Arch Intern Med 1965;115:128–36.
5. Zen Y, Yeh MM. Hepatotoxicity of immune checkpoint inhibitors: a histology study of seven cases in comparison with autoimmune hepatitis and idiosyncratic drug-induced liver injury. Mod Pathol 2018;31(6):965–73.
6. Iacovelli R, Palazzo A, Procopio G, et al. Incidence and relative risk of hepatic toxicity in patients treated with anti-angiogenic tyrosine kinase inhibitors for malignancy. Br J Clin Pharmacol 2014;77(6):929–38.
7. Kok B, Lester ELW, Lee WM, et al. Acute liver failure from tumor necrosis factor-alpha antagonists: report of four cases and literature review. Dig Dis Sci 2018;63(6):1654–66.
8. Taylor SA, Vittorio JM, Martinez M, et al. Anakinra-induced acute liver failure in an adolescent patient with still's disease. Pharmacotherapy 2016;36(1):e1–4.
9. Scully LJ, Clarke D, Barr RJ. Diclofenac induced hepatitis. 3 cases with features of autoimmune chronic active hepatitis. Dig Dis Sci 1993;38(4):744–51.
10. Kleiner DE, Berman D. Pathologic changes in ipilimumab-related hepatitis in patients with metastatic melanoma. Dig Dis Sci 2012;57(8):2233–40.
11. Johncilla M, Misdraji J, Pratt DS, et al. Ipilimumab-associated hepatitis: clinicopathologic characterization in a series of 11 cases. Am J Surg Pathol 2015;39(8):1075–84.
12. Ghabril M, Bonkovsky HL, Kum C, et al. Liver injury from tumor necrosis factor-alpha antagonists: analysis of thirty-four cases. Clin Gastroenterol Hepatol 2013;11(5):558–564 e553.
13. Schattner A, Von der Walde J, Kozak N, et al. Nitrofurantoin-induced immune-mediated lung and liver disease. Am J Med Sci 1999;317(5):336–40.
14. de Boer YS, Kosinski AS, Urban TJ, et al. Features of autoimmune hepatitis in patients with drug-induced liver injury. Clin Gastroenterol Hepatol 2017;15(1):103–112 e102.
15. Black M, Mitchell JR, Zimmerman HJ, et al. Isoniazid-associated hepatitis in 114 patients. Gastroenterology 1975;69(2):289–302.
16. Russo MW, Hoofnagle JH, Gu J, et al. Spectrum of statin hepatotoxicity: experience of the drug-induced liver injury network. Hepatology 2014;60(2):679–86.
17. Zimmerman HJ. Hepatotoxicity: the adverse effects of drugs and other chemicals on the liver. 2nd edition. Philadelphia: Lippincott, Williams & Wilkins; 1999.
18. Mullick FG, Ishak KG. Hepatic injury associated with diphenylhydantoin therapy. A clinicopathologic study of 20 cases. Am J Clin Pathol 1980;74(4):442–52.
19. Vanderstigel M, Zafrani ES, Lejonc JL, et al. Allopurinol hypersensitivity syndrome as a cause of hepatic fibrin-ring granulomas. Gastroenterology 1986;90(1):188–90.
20. Everett J, Srivastava A, Misdraji J. Fibrin ring granulomas in checkpoint inhibitor-induced hepatitis. Am J Surg Pathol 2017;41(1):134–7.
21. Stolz A, Navarro V, Hayashi PH, et al. Severe and protracted cholestasis in 44 young men taking bodybuilding supplements: assessment of genetic, clinical and chemical risk factors. Aliment Pharmacol Ther 2019;49(9):1195–204.
22. Martinez MA, Vuppalanchi R, Fontana RJ, et al. Clinical and histologic features of azithromycin-induced liver injury. Clin Gastroenterol Hepatol 2015;13(2):369–76.e3.

23. Fontana RJ, Hayashi PH, Barnhart H, et al. Persistent liver biochemistry abnormalities are more common in older patients and those with cholestatic drug induced liver injury. Am J Gastroenterol 2015;110(10):1450–9.

24. Medina-Caliz I, Robles-Diaz M, Garcia-Munoz B, et al. Definition and risk factors for chronicity following acute idiosyncratic drug-induced liver injury. J Hepatol 2016;65(3):532–42.

25. Bruno S, Maisonneuve P, Castellana P, et al. Incidence and risk factors for non-alcoholic steatohepatitis: prospective study of 5408 women enrolled in Italian tamoxifen chemoprevention trial. BMJ 2005;330(7497):932.

26. Mori S, Arima N, Ito M, et al. Non-alcoholic steatohepatitis-like pattern in liver biopsy of rheumatoid arthritis patients with persistent transaminitis during low-dose methotrexate treatment. PLoS One 2018;13(8):e0203084.

27. Begriche K, Massart J, Robin MA, et al. Drug-induced toxicity on mitochondria and lipid metabolism: mechanistic diversity and deleterious consequences for the liver. J Hepatol 2011;54(4):773–94.

28. Starko KM, Mullick FG. Hepatic and cerebral pathology findings in children with fatal salicylate intoxication: further evidence for a causal relation between salicylate and Reye's syndrome. Lancet 1983;1(8320):326–9.

29. Fromenty B, Fisch C, Labbe G, et al. Amiodarone inhibits the mitochondrial beta-oxidation of fatty acids and produces microvesicular steatosis of the liver in mice. J Pharmacol Exp Ther 1990;255(3):1371–6.

30. De Bus L, Depuydt P, Libbrecht L, et al. Severe drug-induced liver injury associated with prolonged use of linezolid. J Med Toxicol 2010;6(3):322–6.

31. Scheffner D, Konig S, Rauterberg-Ruland I, et al. Fatal liver failure in 16 children with valproate therapy. Epilepsia 1988;29(5):530–42.

32. Nalbantoglu IL, Tan BR Jr, Linehan DC, et al. Histological features and severity of oxaliplatin-induced liver injury and clinical associations. J Dig Dis 2014;15(10):553–60.

33. Geller SA, Dubinsky MC, Poordad FF, et al. Early hepatic nodular hyperplasia and submicroscopic fibrosis associated with 6-thioguanine therapy in inflammatory bowel disease. Am J Surg Pathol 2004;28(9):1204–11.

34. Czeczok TW, Van Arnam JS, Wood LD, et al. The almost-normal liver biopsy: presentation, clinical associations, and outcome. Am J Surg Pathol 2017;41(9):1247–53.

35. Rutherford A, King LY, Hynan LS, et al. Development of an accurate index for predicting outcomes of patients with acute liver failure. Gastroenterology 2012;143(5):1237–43.

36. Bjornsson E, Kalaitzakis E, Olsson R. The impact of eosinophilia and hepatic necrosis on prognosis in patients with drug-induced liver injury. Aliment Pharmacol Ther 2007;25(12):1411–21.

37. Ndekwe P, Ghabril MS, Zang Y, et al. Substantial hepatic necrosis is prognostic in fulminant liver failure. World J Gastroenterol 2017;23(23):4303–10.

38. Bonkovsky HL, Kleiner DE, Gu J, et al. Clinical presentations and outcomes of bile duct loss caused by drugs and herbal and dietary supplements. Hepatology 2017;65(4):1267–77.

39. Church RJ, Kullak-Ublick GA, Aubrecht J, et al. Candidate biomarkers for the diagnosis and prognosis of drug-induced liver injury: an international collaborative effort. Hepatology 2019;69(2):760–73.

40. Rockey DC, Caldwell SH, Goodman ZD, et al, American Association for the Study of Liver Diseases. Liver biopsy. Hepatology 2009;49(3):1017–44.

41. European Association for the Study of the Liver. EASL clinical practice guidelines: drug-induced liver injury. J Hepatol 2019;70(6):1222–61.

Acute Liver Failure Secondary to Drug-Induced Liver Injury

Maneerat Chayanupatkul, MD[a,b,*], Thomas D. Schiano, MD[c]

KEYWORDS

- Drug-induced acute liver failure • Epidemiology • Clinical presentation • Prognosis
- Liver transplantation

KEY POINTS

- Drug-induced liver injury (DILI), combining both acetaminophen (APAP) and idiosyncratic DILI (iDILI), accounts for more than 50% of all cases of acute liver failure (ALF) in the United States.
- APAP-related ALF presents with a hyperacute liver injury pattern and may progress rapidly to death within a span of 72 hours.
- iDILI-related ALF develops more slowly, over a period of several days to weeks, with less high-grade encephalopathy on initial presentation.
- Approximately 60% of patients with APAP-related ALF survive without liver transplantation, whereas 66% of those with iDILI-related ALF require liver transplantation.
- N-acetylcysteine is recommended for APAP-related ALF and should be considered in iDILI-related ALF, bearing in mind the caveat of unproved overall survival benefit.

INTRODUCTION

Acute liver failure (ALF) is a clinical syndrome characterized by the development of hepatic encephalopathy and coagulopathy (usually defined as international normalized ratio [INR] ≥ 1.5) in the absence of chronic liver disease (CLD), with presumed onset of less than 26 weeks. It is associated with a high mortality rate without liver transplantation. ALF is, however, a rare occurrence, with an estimated incidence in the Western

Disclosure Statement: The authors have nothing to disclose.
[a] Department of Physiology, Chulalongkorn University, Pattayapat Building, 10th Floor, 1873 Rama IV Road, Pathumwan, Bangkok 10330, Thailand; [b] Division of Gastroenterology, Department of Medicine, Chulalongkorn University, Pattayapat Building, 10th Floor, 1873 Rama IV Road, Pathumwan, Bangkok 10330, Thailand; [c] Division of Liver Diseases, Department of Medicine, Recanati/Miller Transplantation Institute, Icahn School of Medicine at Mount Sinai, Icahn Building, 3rd Floor, 1425 Madison Avenue, New York, NY 10029, USA
* Corresponding author. Department of Physiology, Chulalongkorn University, Pattayapat Building, 10th Floor, 1873 Rama IV Road, Pathumwan, Bangkok 10330, Thailand
E-mail address: maneeratc@gmail.com

Clin Liver Dis 24 (2020) 75–87
https://doi.org/10.1016/j.cld.2019.09.005
1089-3261/20/© 2019 Elsevier Inc. All rights reserved.

world of 1.4 to 5.5 cases per million inhabitants per year.[1,2] According to data from the Acute Liver Failure Study Group (ALFSG), drug-induced liver injury (DILI) combining both acetaminophen (APAP) and idiosyncratic DILI (iDILI), accounts for more than 50% of all cases of ALF in the United States (**Fig. 1**).[3] Similarly, a report from the King's College Hospital from 1999 to 2007 showed that 57% and 11% of ALF cases were caused by APAP and iDILI, respectively.[4,5]

EPIDEMIOLOGY OF DRUG-INDUCED ACUTE LIVER FAILURE

In the United States, the proportion of ALF cases related to APAP seem to be on the rise.[6] Data from the ALFSG from 1994 to 1996 and a 13-year study (1983–1995) from the University of Pittsburgh similarly showed that approximately 20% of ALF cases were related to APAP.[7,8] Results from the ALFSG from 1998 to 2001 and from 1998 to 2016 demonstrated that APAP-related ALF was responsible for 39% and 46% of all cases, respectively.[3,9] Despite the decline in hospitalizations related to APAP overdose and a decrease in the sales of APAP after the 1998 regulations on restricting the APAP sale in the United Kingdom, data are conflicting regarding the reduction in mortality and severity of APAP hepatotoxicity in that region.[10,11] Reports from the King's College Hospital, however, have indicated a fall in ALF cases that were associated with APAP, from approximately 70% before 1998 to 57% after 1998.[4,12,13]

The true incidence of iDILI-related ALF is more difficult to determine due to under-reporting and under-recognition. In the United States, iDILI is believed to be responsible for 11% of ALF cases, with the number of iDILI-related ALF and deaths to be 300 to 500 per year.[3,14] A multicenter retrospective study from Spain reported that 17.2% of ALF cases were related to non-APAP drug or toxic reactions, with an estimated incidence of 0.24 cases per million inhabitants per year.[2] The number was higher in a French population-based study, which reported the crude incidence rate of fulminant hepatitis from DILI at 8.2 cases per million inhabitants per year.[15] Among the iDILI cases, the incidence of complementary and alternative medicine (CAM)-induced ALF is rising. The proportion of CAM-related ALF/acute liver injury cases increased from 12.4% from 1998 to 2007 to 21.1% from 2007 to 2015.[16] Moreover, CAM was

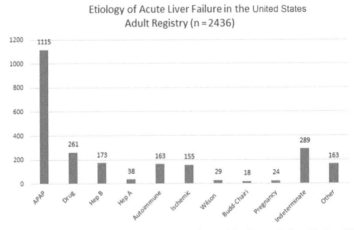

Fig. 1. Etiology of ALF in the United States. Hep, hepatitis. (*From* Tujios SR, Lee WM. Acute liver failure induced by idiosyncratic reaction to drugs: challenges in diagnosis and therapy. *Liver Int* 2018;38(1):6-14; with permission.)

associated with higher transplantation rates and a lower 21-day transplant-free survival compared with prescription drugs.[16]

CLINICAL PRESENTATION AND DIAGNOSTIC APPROACHES

APAP-related ALF occurs as a result of either intentional or unintentional overdose. In contrast to other Western countries, in which suicidal overdose constitutes a majority of APAP-related ALF, unintentional overdose accounts for 50% to 60% of APAP-related ALF in the United States.[6,17,18] Data from a single-center experience showed that patients with suicidal overdoses were more likely to present to the hospital less than 24 hours after the ingestion, had lesser degree of aminotransferase and bilirubin elevations and impaired kidney function, and had lower mortality than those with unintentional overdoses despite lower doses of APAP ingestion.[19] These results were supported by another study from the United Kingdom, which demonstrated that unintentional overdose with APAP-combination products was independently predictive of death or need for liver transplantation.[18] A recent report from the ALFSG indicated that 72% of unintentional APAP overdose were due to combination products (APAP with opioids or diphenhydramine). Patients who overdosed with the APAP/opioid combination were older, predominantly female, and more likely to present with high-grade encephalopathy and had more medical comorbidities than those taking APAP alone. It can be difficult to ascertain whether the encephalopathy is directly related to a failing liver or is related to other concurrently ingested medications, that is, benzodiazepines. In contrast to the studies discussed previously, no mortality differences were found between patients who took APAP alone and those who took combination products.[17]

In patients who present with altered mental status in whom the ingestion history cannot be obtained, certain clinical clues may indicate APAP-related hepatotoxicity, such as female gender and hyperacute liver injury pattern (ALT >3500 IU/L and total bilirubin <5 mg/dL).[20] In cases in which drug exposure cannot be ascertained and APAP levels are not helpful, measuring APAP-CYS adduct levels could aid in the diagnosis of APAP toxicity.[20,21] In comparison to non-APAP ALF, patients with APAP-related ALF are more likely to be younger, female, associated with higher serum ALT and creatinine levels and higher coma grade, and have a higher chance of requiring mechanical ventilation, vasopressor support, or renal replacement therapy as well having a lower serum bilirubin.[22] Differences in clinical characteristics between APAP-related and iDILI-related ALF are presented in **Table 1**.

Clinical features of iDILI-related ALF are different from those of APAP-related ALF. In contrast to the hyperacute presentation of APAP toxicity, iDILI-related ALF develops more slowly, over a period of several days to weeks. According to the ALFSG database and data from the Kaiser Permanente Northern California health care system, modest transaminase elevation with a more pronounced jaundice are more commonly seen in iDILI compared with APAP-related ALF.[23,24] High-grade encephalopathy on initial presentation only occurs in one-third of patients with iDILI-related ALF compared with more than 50% in APAP-related ALF.[22,23] The time from onset of jaundice to hepatic encephalopathy is longest in patients with iDILI-related ALF resulting from dietary/herbal supplements or antimicrobials.[24] Other than fewer medical comorbidities and lower serum alkaline phosphatase levels in patients with CAM-related ALF, patient demographics, presenting symptoms, the onset of jaundice, the pattern of liver injury, coma grade, Model for End-stage Liver Disease (MELD) scores, and median levels of aspartate aminotransferase, alanine aminotransferase (ALT), total bilirubin, and

Table 1
Clinical characteristics of acetaminophen-related acute liver failure versus idiosyncratic drug-induced liver injury–related acute liver failure

	Acetaminophen-Related Acute Liver Failure	Idiosyncratic Drug-Induced Liver Injury–Related Acute Liver Failure
Median age	37	46
Female gender (%)	76	69
Onset of presentation	Hyperacute	Subacute
High-grade encephalopathy (%)	53	36
Pattern of liver chemistry abnormalities	Hyperacute liver injury pattern (ALT >3500 IU/L and total bilirubin <5 mg/dL)	Modest transaminase elevation with a more pronounced jaundice
Specific treatment	NAC	May consider NAC
Spontaneous survival (%)	64.4	25
Transplant rate (%)	8.6	38
1-y post-transplant survival (%)[41]	76	52–82

Adapted from Tujios SR, Lee WM. Acute liver failure induced by idiosyncratic reaction to drugs: challenges in diagnosis and therapy. *Liver Int* 2018;38(1):6-14; with permission.

INR are similar between patients with prescription medication and CAM-related ALF.[16]

Illicit drug use also should be considered as a cause of ALF, especially in young adults. The exact prevalence of illicit drug–related ALF has not been reported in large studies. The examples of illicit drugs that can cause ALF are cocaine, ecstasy, and phencyclidine. Heroin by itself, despite its popularity in the current opioid epidemics, has never been reported to cause ALF.[25] Cocaine-induced hepatotoxicity usually presents with acute hepatocellular injury similar to APAP-induced hepatotoxicity or ischemic hepatitis. Cocaine can cause centrolobular necrosis and fatty changes as a result of direct liver toxicity of cocaine metabolites by cytochrome P450 isoenzymes or by indirect insults related to hepatic ischemia from multiorgan failure or hyperthermia. Spontaneous recovery is expected in approximately 50% of patients.[26,27] Ecstasy and phencyclidine cause ALF by means of severe hyperthermia. Apart from clinical manifestations of ALF, these patients often have hyperthermia, hypotension, rhabdomyolysis, renal failure, and disseminated intravascular coagulation.[25] Liver transplant outcomes in illicit drug–related ALF are limited to case reports only.

Given the lack of diagnostic tests, diagnosis of iDILI-related ALF is based on the temporal association between the drug exposure and clinical presentation, the causal relationship between the pattern of liver injury and the implicated drug, and the exclusion of other causes. The Roussel Uclaf Causality Assessment Method (RUCAM) is a widely used tool in the causality assessment of DILI, which assigns points for clinical, biochemical, serologic, and radiologic features of liver injury and gives an overall score that reflects the likelihood of the implicated drug as a cause of DILI.[28] Using RUCAM is, however, time-consuming and associated with considerable interobserver variation.[29] The list of causative agents that accounts for iDILI-related ALF is shown in **Fig. 2**. Common prescription medications implicated in iDILI-related ALF are isoniazid (18.6% of cases), nitrofurantoin (9.0%), trimethoprim/sulfamethoxazole (6.8%), and

CAUSES OF IDIOSYNCRATIC DRUG–INDUCED ACUTE LIVER
FAILURE

■ Antituberculosis ■ Antibiotics ■ Antiepileptics ■ CAMs ■ NSADs ■ Statins ■ Others

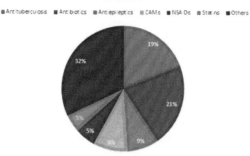

Fig. 2. Causes of idiosyncratic drug-induced ALF by frequency. NSAID, nonsteroidal anti-inflammatory drug. (*From* Makin AJ, Wendon J, Williams R. A 7-year experience of severe acetaminophen-induced hepatotoxicity (1987-1993). *Gastroenterology* 1995;109(6):1907-1916; with permission.)

phenytoin (6.0%), whereas CAM and dietary supplements are responsible for 10.6% of iDILI-related ALF cases.[14] Commonly implicated CAM and dietary supplements in ALF are black cohosh[16] and weight loss products, such as OxyELITE Pro,[30] Hydroxycut,[16] usnic acid,[14] and *Garcinia cambogia* extract.[31] The causative agents associated with iDILI-related ALF are different in the pediatric population, with valproic acid a leading cause (17.0%), followed by isoniazid (8.5%) and propylthiouracil (6.4%).[32]

Liver biopsy is not routinely required if the etiology of ALF can be determined on clinical grounds alone. Transjugular liver biopsy is recommended, however, if there is a suspicion for autoimmune hepatitis, malignant infiltration, or herpes simplex hepatitis.[33] Furthermore, the pattern of liver injury on histology in combination with clinical information may aid in the identification of causative agent(s) in iDILI-related ALF.[34,35] Additionally, certain histologic features confer prognostic value. For example, the presence of extensive hepatocyte necrosis, ductular reaction, fibrosis, microvesicular steatosis, cholangiolar cholestasis, and portal venopathy has been shown to be associated with ALF, death, or liver transplantation within 6 months of DILI onset.[35,36]

Intrinsic CLD may affect drug metabolism and predispose patients with CLD to the development of DILI at a lower dose than in the setting of normal liver function. For instance, patients with nonalcoholic fatty liver disease or alcoholic liver disease are at increased risk of hepatotoxicity from APAP use (even at a therapeutic dose) due to the induction of cytochrome P450 2E1 and the depletion of glutathione (in cases of chronic alcohol use).[37,38] Furthermore, when they develop DILI, patients with pre-existing liver disease are at higher risk of death.[39,40] With abnormal hepatic biomarkers at baseline, clinical features of DILI in patients with CLD may differ from the classic presentation observed in those with normal livers, thus potentially causing a delay in DILI diagnosis. According to a study of acute on chronic liver failure (ACLF) by the Asian Pacific Association for the Study of the Liver research consortium, medications are responsible for the development of ACLF in 6.5% of cases in which anti-tuberculosis therapy and CAM are the most common causes.[41] In this study, ACLF was defined as an acute hepatic insult manifesting as jaundice and coagulopathy, complicated within 4 weeks by the development of ascites and/or encephalopathy in a patient with previously diagnosed or undiagnosed CLD.[42]

CLINICAL OUTCOMES AND PROGNOSIS

The clinical course of APAP-related ALF can evolve rapidly to multiorgan failure and death or spontaneously recover usually within a span of 72 hours.[22] In several studies among listed patients, 24% to 35% died prior to liver transplantation due to significant clinical deterioration and 31% underwent liver transplantation.[6,22,43] Despite more severe clinical features at presentation, approximately 60% of patients with APA-related ALF survive without liver transplantation.[6,22,44] Apart from prognostic scores, summarized later, a recent study showed that serum liver-type fatty acid–binding protein early (day 1) or late (day 3–5) levels could potentially discriminate survivors from nonsurvivors in APAP-related ALF and may improve performance of currently used prognostic models.[45]

In contrast to APAP toxicity, iDILI-related ALF progresses more slowly but carries a worse prognosis. This slower progression may complicate the decision-making process of more rapidly proceeding to transplantation with the hope of spontaneous recovery. Rapid neurologic deterioration and infection may ensue, thus ultimately precluding transplantation. With the aforementioned nature of this condition, patients with iDILI-related ALF are more likely to undergo liver transplantation than those with APAP-related ALF (36% in APAP related vs 66% in iDILI related).[22] Data from the ALFSG from 1998 to 2007 reported that 27.1% of iDILI patients survived without liver transplantation, 42.1% underwent liver transplantation, and 30.8% died.[14] Transplant-free survival in patients with iDILI-related ALF has improved to 41.4% in the recent years.[46] Serum interleukin-17 level has been shown to be associated with high-grade encephalopathy and an independent predictor of death or liver transplantation in non-APAP ALF patients.[47] In patients with CLD, the development of ACLF from drugs is associated with 61% mortality.[41]

Several prognostic scoring systems have been developed to determine the necessity for urgent liver transplantation. The King's College Hospital criteria are one of the oldest and the most widely used prognostic scores. Developed in 1989, the King's College Hospital criteria have been validated in many centers and subjected to several meta-analyses.[8,12,48] They have a high specificity (70%–99%) but low sensitivity (30%–70%) in predicting poor outcomes. These criteria perform better in APAP-related ALF than in non-APAP ALF.[49]

The MELD score is an alternative prognostic scoring system that has recently been shown in a meta-analysis to outperform the King's College Hospital criteria in predicting mortality in patients with non-APAP ALF, with a pooled sensitivity and specificity of 76%, and 73%, respectively.[49] The ALFSG has also developed its own prognostic score to predict 21-day transplant-free survival by incorporating several clinical variables, such as the degree of hepatic encephalopathy, etiology of ALF, vasopressor use, serum bilirubin, and INR.[50] The performance of this model has been shown superior to the prognostic scores discussed previously. The area under the receiver operating characteristic for the ALFSG model was 0.843 compared with 0.717 for MELD score and 0.560 to 0.655 for the King's College Criteria.[50]

With the improvement of medical care in critically ill patients with ALF, overall survival and transplant-free survival rates have improved over time. A longitudinal study over a 16-year period has demonstrated an increase in overall survival and transplant-free survival rates from 58.8% and 32.9% in 1998% to 75.0% and 61.0% in 2013, respectively (**Fig. 3**).[46] The improvement in overall outcomes was apparent for both APAP-related and iDILI-related ALF.

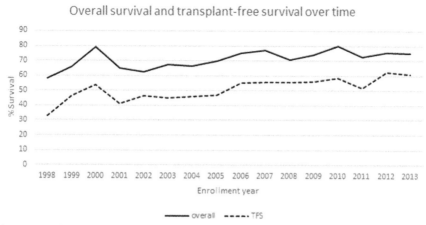

Fig. 3. Overall and liver transplant-free survival (TFS) over time in patients with ALF. (*From* Danan G, Teschke R. RUCAM in drug and herb induced liver injury: The Update. *Int J Mol Sci* 2015;17(1):14; with permission.)

TREATMENT OF DRUG-INDUCED ACUTE LIVER FAILURE

Every patient with ALF should be admitted to an intensive care unit for close monitoring and prompt treatment.[33] Early referral for liver transplant evaluation or expeditious transfer to a liver transplant center is paramount as is contacting the local poison control center. All implicated drugs need to be stopped. Collateral information from family and friends should be obtained with regard to any prescription medications, over-the-counter products, and use of alcohol and illicit drugs.

N-acetylcysteine (NAC) has been shown to be safe and effective in the treatment of APAP-related ALF even when administered 48 hours or more after the ingestion, and its use is endorsed by the American Association for the Study of Liver Diseases.[33,51,52] NAC works by replenishing glutathione stores, increasing oxygen delivery and consumption, and reducing inflammatory cytokine production.[47,53] The benefit of NAC in non-APAP ALF, however, has been a subject of debate. A prospective trial demonstrated a transplant-free survival benefit in non-APAP ALF patients with coma grades I to II who received NAC but not in those with coma grades III to IV. The overall survival and transplantation rate were not different between the NAC and placebo groups. In a subgroup of patients with iDILI-related ALF, transplant-free survival improved from 27% in placebo to 58% in NAC group.[54] A meta-analysis of 4 prospective trials showed an improvement in transplant-free survival and post-transplant survival in non-APAP ALF patients who received NAC but again did not show any benefit in overall survival.[55] Due to its excellent safety profile, NAC may be considered in iDILI-related ALF, bearing in mind the caveat that it may not improve overall survival.

Despite its popularity as a treatment of DILI, corticosteroids have never been proved beneficial in iDILI-related ALF.[56] A randomized controlled trial evaluating the effect of hydrocortisone in patients with ALF did not show a survival benefit in those who received hydrocortisone.[57] Data from the ALFSG registry between 1998 and 2007 demonstrated that corticosteroid use did not improve overall survival and spontaneous survival in drug-induced (DI)-ALF patients. Corticosteroid use was associated with lower overall survival in patients with MELD greater than 40.[58] Corticosteroid administration is, therefore, not recommended in patients with iDILI-related ALF.

LIVER TRANSPLANTATION FOR DRUG-INDUCED ACUTE LIVER FAILURE

With the advent of liver transplantation, the mortality rate in patients with ALF has dropped significantly. Nevertheless, these patients are still at risk for early death or graft loss after liver transplantation, especially during the first year. An analysis of the United Network for Organ Sharing (UNOS) database from 1987 to 2006 showed that 1-year estimated survival probabilities of patients transplanted for DI-ALF were 76%, 82%, 52%, 82%, and 79% for APAP, antituberculosis drugs, antiepileptics, antibiotics, and others, respectively. The survival rates were similar between adult and pediatric patients with the exception of pediatric patients transplanted for antiepileptic-induced ALF who had significantly higher post-transplant mortality. This finding might be related to the higher degree of encephalopathy precipitated by valproic-induced hyperammonemia, which adversely affects post-transplant outcomes. The overall survival between APAP-related and non-APAP-related ALF were similar, and the independent pretransplant predictors of death after liver transplantation were DI-ALF due to antiepileptic drugs at age less than 18, being on life support, and high serum creatinine.[32]

In contrast to the US report, data from the European Liver Transplant Registry database (January 1988–June 2009) demonstrated the 1-year, 3-year, 5-year, and 10-year patient survival rates in those transplanted for ALF to be 74%, 70%, 68%, 63%, respectively, with APAP-related ALF as an independent predictor of death or graft loss (relative risk 1.24; 95% CI, 1.03–1.51). In this study, patients who underwent liver transplantation for APAP-related ALF had a 10-times higher rate of social problems as a cause of death or graft loss than other etiologies. Suicide was responsible for a majority of this group of deaths.[59] These results suggest that psychosocial support is important for patients transplanted for APAP-related ALF in order to decrease graft loss and death post-transplantation. APAP-related ALF from a suicidal attempt is, however, not a contraindication for liver transplantation because other studies have shown that repeat suicide attempts actually rarely occur post–liver transplant in patients with APAP-related ALF with similar long-term outcomes and rates of compliance with clinic visits and immunosuppression medication adherence in patients transplanted for APAP-related ALF when compared with those transplanted for CLD.[60–62] This decreased repeat suicide rate may be related to patients being followed in a more structured environment with regimented social work and psychiatric involvement.

Living donor liver transplantation (LDLT) may reduce waiting time for patients with ALF by providing alternative sources of grafts and is particularly important in some parts of the world where a majority of transplanted patients undergo LDLT. In experienced centers, the post-transplant outcomes of LDLT for ALF are comparable to those of deceased donor liver transplantation.[63–65] There are certain issues to consider, however, when using LDLT for patients with ALF. The donor evaluation needs to be expedited in the time-constrained setting of ALF so there might not be sufficient time to assess spontaneous donor's willingness and for thorough medical and ethical evaluation by the transplant teams. The expedited process could lead to increased donor postoperative medical or psychosocial problems.

Despite the improvement in the overall care of liver transplant recipients, the post-transplant mortality remains higher in patients transplanted for ALF than in those patients transplanted for CLD.[66] Several risk factors associated with increased risk of post-transplant mortality, such as the requirement for pretransplant renal support, the use of segmental grafts, and the use of ABO-incompatible grafts, may be seen more frequently in patients transplanted for ALF.[59,66,67] Due to the urgent need for liver transplantation, the high-risk grafts (such as split livers, auxiliary livers, and more extended criteria donors) might be used in patients with ALF, which by itself is a risk factor for post-transplant mortality.[68] Another possible reason for poorer outcomes is a higher rate of acute rejection. A report from a single-center study showed that ALF as an indication for liver transplantation was an independent predictor for the development of moderate to severe acute cellular rejection in the first year after transplant.[69] Rejection rates do not appear to differ between APAP related ALF and iDILI-related ALF.[59] According to the UNOS database, the most common causes of death post-transplant are infection, followed by neurologic complications and multiorgan failure, which are the things patients with ALF are at higher risk for and might even go into transplant with.[70] Choosing the appropriate candidates to undergo liver transplantation and excellent postoperative care are keys to improve outcomes after liver transplantation in ALF patients.

SUMMARY

DILI (APAP and idiosyncratic drugs combined) is the most common cause of ALF in the Western countries. Without liver transplantation, the mortality rate for ALF can be up to 80%. APAP-related ALF is associated with rapid progression but fortunately with a higher chance of spontaneous survival compared with with iDILI-related ALF that evolves more slowly but carries a worse prognosis. NAC is recommended for the treatment of APAP-related ALF but also can be considered in iDILI-related ALF with a questionable benefit on overall survival. Several prognostic scoring systems have been developed to aid clinicians in selecting patients who require urgent liver transplantation. Patients who received liver transplantation for ALF are at risk for lower graft and patient survival and should be closely followed, especially in the social aspect of APAP-related ALF.

REFERENCES

1. Bower WA, Johns M, Margolis HS, et al. Population-based surveillance for acute liver failure. Am J Gastroenterol 2007;102(11):2459–63.
2. Escorsell A, Mas A, de la Mata M. Acute liver failure in Spain: analysis of 267 cases. Liver Transpl 2007;13(10):1389–95.
3. Tujios SR, Lee WM. Acute liver failure induced by idiosyncratic reaction to drugs: challenges in diagnosis and therapy. Liver Int 2018;38(1):6–14.
4. Bernal W, Auzinger G, Wendon J. Prognostic utility of the bilirubin lactate and etiology score. Clin Gastroenterol Hepatol 2009;7(2):249.
5. Bernal W, Auzinger G, Dhawan A, et al. Acute liver failure. Lancet 2010; 376(9736):190–201.
6. Larson AM, Polson J, Fontana RJ, et al. Acetaminophen-induced acute liver failure: results of a United States multicenter, prospective study. Hepatology 2005; 42(6):1364–72.
7. Schiodt FV, Atillasoy E, Shakil AO, et al. Etiology and outcome for 295 patients with acute liver failure in the United States. Liver Transpl Surg 1999;5(1):29–34.
8. Shakil AO, Kramer D, Mazariegos GV, et al. Acute liver failure: clinical features, outcome analysis, and applicability of prognostic criteria. Liver Transpl 2000; 6(2):163–9.
9. Ostapowicz G, Fontana RJ, Schiodt FV, et al. Results of a prospective study of acute liver failure at 17 tertiary care centers in the United States. Ann Intern Med 2002;137(12):947–54.

10. Morgan O, Majeed A. Restricting paracetamol in the United Kingdom to reduce poisoning: a systematic review. J Public Health (Oxf) 2005;27(1):12–8.
11. Sheen CL, Dillon JF, Bateman DN, et al. Paracetamol pack size restriction: the impact on paracetamol poisoning and the over-the-counter supply of paracetamol, aspirin and ibuprofen. Pharmacoepidemiol Drug Saf 2002;11(4):329–31.
12. O'Grady JG, Alexander GJ, Hayllar KM, et al. Early indicators of prognosis in fulminant hepatic failure. Gastroenterology 1989;97(2):439–45.
13. Makin AJ, Wendon J, Williams R. A 7-year experience of severe acetaminophen-induced hepatotoxicity (1987-1993). Gastroenterology 1995;109(6):1907–16.
14. Reuben A, Koch DG, Lee WM. Drug-induced acute liver failure: results of a U.S. multicenter, prospective study. Hepatology 2010;52(6):2065–76.
15. Sgro C, Clinard F, Ouazir K, et al. Incidence of drug-induced hepatic injuries: a French population-based study. Hepatology 2002;36(2):451–5.
16. Hillman L, Gottfried M, Whitsett M, et al. Clinical features and outcomes of complementary and alternative medicine induced acute liver failure and injury. Am J Gastroenterol 2016;111(7):958–65.
17. Serper M, Wolf MS, Parikh NA, et al. Risk factors, clinical presentation, and outcomes in overdose with acetaminophen alone or with combination products: results from the acute liver failure study group. J Clin Gastroenterol 2016;50(1):85–91.
18. Craig DGN, Bates CM, Davidson JS, et al. Overdose pattern and outcome in paracetamol-induced acute severe hepatotoxicity. Br J Clin Pharmacol 2011;71(2):273–82.
19. Schiødt FV, Rochling FA, Casey DL, et al. Acetaminophen toxicity in an urban county hospital. N Engl J Med 1997;337(16):1112–8.
20. Khandelwal N, James LP, Sanders C, et al. Unrecognized acetaminophen toxicity as a cause of indeterminate acute liver failure. Hepatology 2011;53(2):567–76.
21. Ganger DR, Rule J, Rakela J, et al. Acute liver failure of indeterminate etiology: a comprehensive systematic approach by an expert committee to establish causality. Am J Gastroenterol 2018;113(9):1319–28.
22. Reddy KR, Ellerbe C, Schilsky M, et al. Determinants of outcome among patients with acute liver failure listed for liver transplantation in the United States. Liver Transpl 2016;22(4):505–15.
23. Lee WM. Drug-induced acute liver failure. Clin Liver Dis 2013;17(4):575–viii.
24. Goldberg DS, Forde KA, Carbonari DM, et al. Population-representative incidence of drug-induced acute liver failure based on an analysis of an integrated health care system. Gastroenterology 2015;148(7):1353–61.e3.
25. Riordan SM, Williams R. Liver disease due to illicit substance use. Addict Biol 1998;3:47–53.
26. Kanel GC, Cassidy W, Shuster L, et al. Cocaine-induced liver cell injury: comparison of morphological features in man and in experimental models. Hepatology 1990;11(4):646–51.
27. Wanless IR, Dore S, Gopinath N, et al. Histopathology of cocaine hepatotoxicity. Report of four patients. Gastroenterology 1990;98(2):497–501.
28. Danan G, Teschke R. RUCAM in drug and herb induced liver injury: the Update. Int J Mol Sci 2015;17(1):14.
29. Rockey DC, Seeff LB, Rochon J, et al. Causality assessment in drug-induced liver injury using a structured expert opinion process: comparison to the Roussel-Uclaf causality assessment method. Hepatology 2010;51(6):2117–26.
30. Navarro VJ, Khan I, Bjornsson E, et al. Liver injury from herbal and dietary supplements. Hepatology 2017;65(1):363–73.

31. Lunsford KE, Bodzin AS, Reino DC, et al. Dangerous dietary supplements: Garcinia cambogia-associated hepatic failure requiring transplantation. World J Gastroenterol 2016;22(45):10071–6.
32. Mindikoglu AL, Magder LS, Regev A. Outcome of liver transplantation for drug-induced acute liver failure in the United States: analysis of the United Network for Organ Sharing database. Liver Transpl 2009;15(7):719–29.
33. Lee WM, Stravitz RT, Larson AM. AASLD position paper: the management of acute liver failure: Update 2011. Hepatology 2011;55:1–22.
34. Kleiner DE. Liver histology in the diagnosis and prognosis of drug-induced liver injury. Clin Liver Dis 2014;4(1):12–6.
35. Kleiner DE, Chalasani NP, Lee WM, et al. Hepatic histological findings in suspected drug-induced liver injury: systematic evaluation and clinical associations. Hepatology 2014;59(2):661–70.
36. Katoonizadeh A, Nevens F, Verslype C, et al. Liver regeneration in acute severe liver impairment: a clinicopathological correlation study. Liver Int 2006;26(10):1225–33.
37. Teschke R, Danan G. Drug-induced liver injury: is chronic liver disease a risk factor and a clinical issue? Expert Opin Drug Metab Toxicol 2017;13(4):425–38.
38. Yaghi C, Assaf A. Acetaminophen toxicity at therapeutic doses. Inter Med Rev 2017;3(11):1–13.
39. Chalasani N, Bonkovsky HL, Fontana R, et al. Features and outcomes of 899 patients with drug-induced liver injury: the DILIN prospective study. Gastroenterology 2015;148(7):1340–52.e7.
40. Chalasani N, Regev A. Drug-induced liver injury in patients with preexisting chronic liver disease in drug development: how to identify and manage? Gastroenterology 2016;151(6):1046–51.
41. Devarbhavi H, Choudhury AK, Reddy VV, et al. Acute on chronic liver failure secondary to drugs: causes, outcome and predictors of mortality. J Hepatol 2016;64(2):S232.
42. Sarin SK, Kumar A, Almeida JA, et al. Acute-on-chronic liver failure: consensus recommendations of the Asian Pacific Association for the study of the liver (APASL). Hepatol Int 2009;3(1):269–82.
43. Bernal W, Wendon J, Rela M, et al. Use and outcome of liver transplantation in acetaminophen-induced acute liver failure. Hepatology 1998;27(4):1050–5.
44. Bretherick AD, Craig DGN, Masterton G, et al. Acute liver failure in Scotland between 1992 and 2009; incidence, aetiology and outcome. QJM 2011;104(11):945–56.
45. Karvellas CJ, Speiser JL, Tremblay M, et al. Elevated FABP1 serum levels are associated with poorer survival in acetaminophen-induced acute liver failure. Hepatology 2017;65(3):938–49.
46. Reuben A, Tillman H, Fontana RJ, et al. Outcomes in adults with acute liver failure between 1998 and 2013: an observational cohort study. Ann Intern Med 2016;164(11):724–32.
47. Stravitz RT, Sanyal AJ, Reisch J, et al. Effects of N-acetylcysteine on cytokines in non-acetaminophen acute liver failure: potential mechanism of improvement in transplant-free survival. Liver Int 2013;33(9):1324–31.
48. O'Grady J. Timing and benefit of liver transplantation in acute liver failure. J Hepatol 2014;60(3):663–70.
49. McPhail MJ, Farne H, Senvar N, et al. Ability of King's College criteria and model for end-stage liver disease scores to predict mortality of patients with acute liver failure: a meta-analysis. Clin Gastroenterol Hepatol 2016;14(4):516–25.

50. Koch DG, Tillman H, Durkalski V, et al. Development of a model to predict transplant-free survival of patients with acute liver failure. Clin Gastroenterol Hepatol 2016;14(8):1199–206.e2.

51. Harrison PM, Keays R, Bray GP, et al. Improved outcome of paracetamol-induced fulminant hepatic failure by late administration of acetylcysteine. Lancet 1990; 335(8705):1572–3.

52. Keays R, Harrison PM, Wendon JA, et al. Intravenous acetylcysteine in paracetamol induced fulminant hepatic failure: a prospective controlled trial. BMJ 1991; 303(6809):1026–9.

53. Harrison PM, Wendon JA, Gimson AE, et al. Improvement by acetylcysteine of hemodynamics and oxygen transport in fulminant hepatic failure. N Engl J Med 1991;324(26):1852–7.

54. Lee WM, Hynan LS, Rossaro L, et al. Intravenous N-acetylcysteine improves transplant-free survival in early stage non-acetaminophen acute liver failure. Gastroenterology 2009;137(3):856–64, 864.e1.

55. Hu J, Zhang Q, Ren X, et al. Efficacy and safety of acetylcysteine in "non-acetaminophen" acute liver failure: a meta-analysis of prospective clinical trials. Clin Res Hepatol Gastroenterol 2015;39(5):594–9.

56. Hu PF, Xie WF. Corticosteroid therapy in drug-induced liver injury: pros and cons. J Dig Dis 2019;20(3):122–6.

57. Rakela J, Mosley JW, Edwards VM, et al. A double-blinded, randomized trial of hydrocortisone in acute hepatic failure. The Acute Hepatic Failure Study Group. Dig Dis Sci 1991;36(9):1223–8.

58. Karkhanis J, Verna EC, Chang MS, et al. Steroid use in acute liver failure. Hepatology 2014;59(2):612–21.

59. Germani G, Theocharidou E, Adam R, et al. Liver transplantation for acute liver failure in Europe: outcomes over 20 years from the ELTR database. J Hepatol 2012;57(2):288–96.

60. Cooper SC, Aldridge RC, Shah T, et al. Outcomes of liver transplantation for paracetamol (acetaminophen)-induced hepatic failure. Liver Transpl 2009;15(10): 1351–7.

61. Karvellas CJ, Safinia N, Auzinger G, et al. Medical and psychiatric outcomes for patients transplanted for acetaminophen-induced acute liver failure: a case-control study. Liver Int 2010;30(6):826–33.

62. Rhodes R, Aggarwal S, Schiano TD. Overdose with suicidal intent: ethical considerations for liver transplant programs. Liver Transpl 2011;17(9):1111–6.

63. Yamashiki N, Sugawara Y, Tamura S, et al. Outcomes after living donor liver transplantation for acute liver failure in Japan: results of a nationwide survey. Liver Transpl 2012;18(9):1069–77.

64. Campsen J, Blei AT, Emond JC, et al. Outcomes of living donor liver transplantation for acute liver failure: the adult-to-adult living donor liver transplantation cohort study. Liver Transpl 2008;14(9):1273–80.

65. Choudhary NS, Saigal S, Saraf N, et al. Good outcome of living donor liver transplantation in drug-induced acute liver failure: a single-center experience. Clin Transplant 2017;31(3):e12907.

66. Dawwas MF, Gimson AE, Lewsey JD, et al. Survival after liver transplantation in the United Kingdom and Ireland compared with the United States. Gut 2007; 56(11):1606–13.

67. Transplant RCoSaNBa. UK liver transplant audit November 2012. Available at: https://www.rcseng.ac.uk/surgeons/research/surgical-research/docs/liver-transplant-auditreport-2012. Accessed March 19, 2019.

68. Bernal W, Cross TJ, Auzinger G, et al. Outcome after wait-listing for emergency liver transplantation in acute liver failure: a single centre experience. J Hepatol 2009;50(2):306–13.
69. Au KP, Chan SC, Chok KS, et al. Clinical factors affecting rejection rates in liver transplantation. Hepatobiliary Pancreat Dis Int 2015;14(4):367–73.
70. Barshes NR, Lee TC, Balkrishnan R, et al. Risk stratification of adult patients undergoing orthotopic liver transplantation for fulminant hepatic failure. Transplantation 2006;81(2):195–201.

Drug-Induced Liver Injury in the Setting of Chronic Liver Disease

Nicholas A. Hoppmann, MD*, Meagan E. Gray, MD,
Brendan M. McGuire, MD, MS

KEYWORDS

- Drug-induced liver injury • Chronic liver disease • Hepatotoxicity
- Acute-on-chronic liver failure

KEY POINTS

- Drug-induced liver injury (DILI) in the setting of chronic liver disease (CLD) is poorly understood.
- Studies favor CLD as a risk factor for DILI, although more investigation needs to be done in this area.
- Without objective biomarkers, diagnosis of DILI in CLD requires good clinical judgment and high index of suspicion.
- Management of DILI in CLD hinges on identifying and stopping the offending agents as well as early consultation with a liver transplant center.
- Prognosis is often worse in patients with underlying liver disease and DILI.

INTRODUCTION

Drug-induced liver injury (DILI) is one of the leading causes of acute liver failure in the United States, but remains a rare clinical event in patients with chronic liver disease. Although population-based studies have estimated the annual incidence of DILI between 14 and 19 per 100,000 inhabitants,[1,2] only a small percentage of these cases have occurred in patients with preexisting liver disease. Although previously not thought to be a risk factor for DILI, certain causes of chronic liver disease (CLD) may predispose patients to pharmaceutical hepatotoxicity.

At present, diagnosis relies on extensive patient history as well as exclusion of other causes of liver injury, which can prove challenging in patients with CLD given that flares of underlying liver disease can mimic DILI. Existing diagnostic tools and

Disclosure: The authors have nothing to disclose.
Division of Gastroenterology and Hepatology, University of Alabama at Birmingham, 1720 2nd Ave South, Birmingham AL 35294-0012, USA
* Corresponding author.
E-mail address: nhoppmann@uabmc.edu

Clin Liver Dis 24 (2020) 89–106
https://doi.org/10.1016/j.cld.2019.09.006
1089-3261/20/© 2019 Elsevier Inc. All rights reserved.

liver.theclinics.com

prognostic methods have not been evaluated in the setting of CLD except for patients who develop acute-on-chronic liver failure (ACLF). When DILI does occur in patients with CLD, outcomes tend to be worse.

With the incidence of CLD increasing, as well as the exponential increase in pharmaceutical drugs, there is great concern for increasing rates of DILI in patients with CLD.[3,4] This concern places increased pressure on medical providers to know the hepatotoxic risks of medications prescribed to this subgroup of patients.

DEFINITION

DILI is defined as a liver injury caused by various medications, herbs, or other xenobiotics, leading to abnormalities in liver tests or liver dysfunction after reasonable exclusion of other causes.[5] There is no separate definition of DILI in patients with CLD and therefore current definitions are the same as those for patients without CLD. The most common causes of CLD are shown in **Box 1**. In the United States, nonalcoholic fatty liver disease (NAFLD), alcohol-related liver disease, and chronic hepatitis B and C make up the most common causes.[3]

DILI can be categorized as intrinsic or idiosyncratic. Intrinsic DILI is caused by agents with predictable dose-related hepatotoxicity, such as acetaminophen. Idiosyncratic DILI refers to injury caused by agents without a predictable level of hepatotoxicity. The cause of idiosyncratic DILI is unclear but several mechanisms have been proposed, including reactive metabolites, immunoallergic reactions, and genetic factors such as variations in drug metabolism.[6–10] DILI cases can also be categorized as mild, moderate, severe, or fatal based on the DILI severity classification, which takes into account laboratory criteria including bilirubin, alkaline phosphatase (AP), alanine aminotransferase (ALT), aspartate aminotransferase (AST), and international normalized ratio (INR), as well as clinical criteria including ascites, encephalopathy, duration of injury, and presence of other organ failure.[11]

There are 3 standard definitions for liver injury, drug induced or otherwise: (1) increases of ALT or AST level more than 5 times the upper limit of normal (ULN) or AP level more than 2 times the ULN on 2 separate occasions, (2) total bilirubin level greater than 2.5 mg/dL along with increases in AST or ALT or AP level, or (3) INR greater than 1.5 with increased AST, ALT, or AP level.[6] A separate definition was previously proposed with stricter guidelines; however, this has not been widely adopted.[12] Variations in definitions among different studies have complicated interpretation of their respective findings. When evaluating biochemical injury for DILI in the setting of CLD, most studies recommend comparison with baseline values

---

Box 1
Common causes of chronic liver disease

Chronic viral hepatitis
  Chronic hepatitis B
  Chronic hepatitis C

Nonalcoholic fatty liver disease

Alcoholic liver disease

Autoimmune hepatitis

Chronic cholestatic disorders
  Primary biliary cholangitis
  Primary sclerosing cholangitis

(which are often increased) instead of the ULN, although no standardized increases have been proposed.[2,6]

The pattern of injury can be characterized as hepatocellular, cholestatic, or mixed. The R value is defined as the ratio of ALT to AP, with the ALT and AP expressed as multiples of the ULN. The R value can be used to differentiate between these patterns with R value greater than or equal to 5 indicating hepatocellular injury, R value less than or equal to 2 cholestatic, and R value between 2 and 5 classified as mixed.[6,7,10]

EPIDEMIOLOGY

Idiosyncratic DILI is rare and occurs in less than 1 per 10,000 to 1 per 100,000 individuals, with only a small percentage of these cases occurring in patients with CLD.[7,13] The incidence of DILI in patients with preexisting CLD is estimated to be between 4% and 14% of all DILI cases, based on large population-based studies shown in **Table 1**.[1,2,14–16] Differences in the reported data have made comparisons challenging. Only the Drug-Induced Liver Injury Network (DILIN) prospective registry in the United States has provided detailed information regarding the cause of CLD in patients with DILI. Out of 899 total patients with DILI in this registry, 89 (10%) had evidence of CLD. Thirty-six patients had chronic hepatitis C, with the remaining 47 having either NAFLD or unknown cause of chronically increased liver tests.

RISK FACTORS

The growing prevalence of CLD, particularly NAFLD,[17] has raised concerns for increasing opportunities for DILI to occur in the setting of underlying liver disease. Identifying risk factors that predispose patients toward DILI is challenging because of its low incidence.[10,13] Previously, there was no evidence to support CLD as a risk factor for developing DILI[18]; however, more recent studies have raised concern for increased hepatotoxicity in certain settings. One such scenario includes treatment of tuberculosis or human immunodeficiency virus (HIV) in patients with viral hepatitis.[2,4,6,7,19–23] Most of these studies failed to control for expected fluctuations of liver tests in viral hepatitis and therefore it is not clear whether these cases represented true drug-induced hepatotoxicity.[23] Two studies have shown that patients with underlying liver disease are more likely to develop DILI.[24,25] One of these found that patients with NAFLD were 3 times as likely to develop DILI with an odds ratio of 3.95 compared with those with chronic hepatitis C.[24] All of the patients who developed DILI in this cohort

Table 1		
Population-based studies of drug-induced liver injury		
Study	Total Number of Patients	Patients with CLD
Sgro et al,[1] 2002 France	34	Number not reported
Björnsson et al,[2] 2013 Iceland	96	4 (4.1%)
Chalasani et al,[16] 2015 United States	899	89 (10%)[c]
De Valle et al,[15] 2006 Sweden	77	11 (14%)[a]
Andrade et al,[14] 2005 Spain	446	22 (4.9%)[b]

[a] Autoimmune hepatitis (n = 6), nonalcoholic steatohepatitis (n = 2), alcoholic liver disease (n = 1), cryptogenic (n = 1), primary biliary cholangitis/primary sclerosing cholangitis (n = 1).
[b] Cirrhosis (n = 8), alcoholic hepatitis (n = 3).
[c] Patients with hepatitis C virus (n = 36), hepatitis B virus (n = 6), NAFLD or unexplained abnormal liver function test (n = 47).

also had an increased waist/hip ratio, raising the question of the role of central adiposity, or NAFLD as a risk factor in the development of DILI. In a separate study, patients with unexplained increases in ALT levels (>45 units per liter) had a 6-fold increased risk for DILI compared with those without suspected underlying liver disease (P<.001).[25] These studies strongly support the suspicion that CLD is a risk factor for DILI.

Among the 899 patients included in the DILIN study, no significant differences were found between patients with and without CLD regarding age at presentation, gender, body mass index, prior drug allergies, or racial distribution. However, patients with DILI and CLD were more likely to be diabetic.[16]

PRESENTATION

Clinical features among patients with CLD who develop DILI are similar to those without CLD. Presenting signs and symptoms are variable and nonspecific, including lethargy, nausea, vomiting, abdominal pain, and anorexia. They may have jaundice, pruritus, and dark urine. Jaundice is present in approximately 70% of patients with CLD who develop DILI based on the DILIN data, which is similar to the rate of jaundice in patients without CLD.[16] This figure may overestimate rates of jaundice in cases of DILI in the general population given the severity of patients transferred to tertiary care centers in the DILIN network.

Biochemically, patients who develop DILI with and without CLD also present similarly, with hepatocellular injury being the most common (45%–54%), followed by cholestatic (31%–40%) and mixed (13%–15%) injury.[15,16] Patients with CLD tend to have lower peak ALT and AP levels compared with those without CLD; however, INR values are similar.[16] Baseline liver tests should be considered in patients with CLD during evaluation for possible DILI as opposed to ULN.

EVALUATION AND DIAGNOSIS

DILI remains a diagnosis of exclusion, which can be challenging in CLD because flares of underlying liver disease can mimic DILI, including viral, autoimmune, and alcohol-related liver disease.[3,13,26] Diagnosis in the setting of CLD requires a high index of suspicion. Patient history can be misleading because some patients are unaware of underlying liver disease.[27] Careful attention should be paid to alcohol use, new medications, herbal or dietary supplements (HDSs), comorbidities, and current clinical status. **Table 2** reviews the recommended laboratory evaluation that should be obtained during evaluation of DILI to exclude other potential causes of increased liver tests.[3,7,28]

Causality is an essential component in the diagnosis of DILI. Several tools have been proposed for determining causality of an offending agent, although none have been evaluated in patients with CLD. The most commonly used tool is the Rousel-Uclaf Causality Assessment Method (RUCAM), which involves 7 elements: (1) time of onset from beginning the drug, (2) course after drug cessation, (3) risk factors (age, alcohol use, pregnancy), (4) concomitant drug use, (5) exclusion of other causes of liver injury, (6) previous information on hepatotoxicity of the drug, and (7) response to readministration.[3,27] Scores from each section are tallied and can categorize DILI as highly probable (>8), probable (6–8), possible (3–5), unlikely (1 or 2), or excluded (≤0).[6,29,30] RUCAM has been criticized as cumbersome, with ambiguity of certain components limiting its clinical use.[6,27,29–31] Studies have found RUCAM to have poor reproducibility, even when repeated by the same reviewers, and it is therefore not recommended for isolated use when assessing casualty of DILI.[3,27,32] Using the RUCAM as well

Table 2
Recommended laboratory evaluation in patients with suspected drug-induced liver injury

Possible Cause of Liver Injury	Laboratory Data
Wilson disease	Low ceruloplasmin level AP/bilirubin ratio <4
Viral Hepatitis	
Hepatitis A	Anti–hepatitis A virus IgM
Hepatitis B	Hepatitis B surface antigen Hepatitis B core antibody, total and IgM HBV DNA
Hepatitis C	Hepatitis C antibody (total) HCV RNA
Hepatitis D	Hepatitis D antibody (total) HDV RNA
Epstein-Barr	EBV IgM EBV DNA
If Immunosuppressed/Pregnant:	
CMV	CMV IgM CMV DNA
Herpes Simplex	HSV 1 and 2 IgM HSV 1 and 2 DNA quantification
Hepatitis E	Anti-HEV IgM
Autoimmune hepatitis	Antinuclear antibody Anti–smooth muscle antibody Total IgG level
Alcoholic hepatitis	Total bilirubin >3 mg/dL ALT and AST >1.5 × ULN but <400 units/L AST/ALT ratio >1.5 Increased phosphatidylethanol level Leukocytosis/neutrophilia Increased mean corpuscular volume
Biliary obstruction	Abdominal ultrasonography Magnetic resonance cholangiopancreatography
Vascular/Budd-Chiari	Abdominal ultrasonography with Doppler

Abbreviations: CMV, cytomegalovirus; EBV, Epstein-Barr virus; HBV, hepatitis B virus; HCV, hepatitis C virus; HDV, hepatitis D virus; HEV, hepatitis E virus; HSV, herpes simplex virus; Ig, immunoglobulin.

as a causality committee, the DILIN group found fewer cases of highly probable DILI in patients with preexisting liver disease compared with those without (17% vs 27%; $P = .009$), likely reflecting the difficulty of differentiating DILI from flares of CLD in this group.[16]

Latency refers to the time of onset of DILI following administration of the offending agent. DILI usually occurs in the first 6 months of exposure, although some cases have been fatal after only a few days. Nitrofurantoin, minocycline, and HDSs often have longer latency periods.[3] There was no statistical difference in latency among patients with or without CLD in the DILIN report, with median onset 34 to 36 days among both groups.[16]

The period after drug cessation, often called the washout or dechallenge, can also be helpful in confirming DILI. Experts suggest consideration of alternative causes of liver injury if peak ALT level has not declined by 50% in 30 days, although others recommend a 60-day cutoff.[3,30,32,33] Overall, cholestatic DILI resolves more slowly, and 180 days is recommended as a threshold for assessing resolution.[3] From the DILIN data, ALT levels normalize quicker in patients with mixed DILI (59 days), compared with hepatocellular (79 days) and cholestatic (113 days) injury. AP levels normalize fastest in patients with hepatocellular injury (48 days), compared with mixed (90 days) and cholestatic (183 days) DILI. There was no significant difference in time to improvement of liver tests found between patients with and without CLD.[16]

Many medications as well as HDSs known to cause hepatotoxicity have a signature with regard to their latency and pattern of biochemical injury that can aid in assessing causality.[3,7] HDS are an important category that should be considered and investigated in every patient with suspected DILI. These agents are marketed without approval from the US Food and Drug Administration (FDA), which means ingredients and concentrations can have significant variations.[6] LiverTox (https://livertox.nlm.nih. gov) is an online database providing up-to-date information on the diagnosis, cause, frequency, pattern, and management of hepatotoxicity related to prescription and nonprescription medications and supplements.[34] Each recorded substance has information regarding the pharmacology of the drug, its association with prior hepatotoxicity, mechanism of injury (if known), as well as outcomes and management. Prior case reports submitted to LiverTox are included with a timeline of the patient's clinical course, laboratory data, and time to resolution. References for additional published cases are also provided. Although presentations can differ from prior reported cases, LiverTox is a valuable tool in assessing DILI causality. It is also notable that up to 20% of DILI cases can be attributed to more than 1 agent.[6] Ultimately, despite these tools, expert opinion is still considered the gold standard for the diagnosis of DILI in patients both with and without CLD. Good clinical judgment and a high index of suspicion are crucial.

UNIQUE ISSUES ON SPECIFIC DRUGS OR CLASSES OF DRUGS

The low incidence of DILI and exclusion of patients with CLD in clinical trials means the safety of many medications in CLD is uncertain.[7,10,35] Changes in the volume of distribution and/or hepatic blood flow can interfere with drug metabolism in patients with compensated and decompensated cirrhosis.[36] Antibiotics and antiepileptics remain the most common causes, accounting for more than 60% of all DILI cases both with and without CLD.[3,6,16] Other common causes include HDSs, cardiovascular agents, and antineoplastic agents; all of these are implicated at a similar frequency between patients with and without underlying liver disease.

Isoniazid, azithromycin, amoxicillin-clavulanate, and nitrofurantoin were the top agents reported to cause DILI in patients with CLD in the DILIN database.[16] Azithromycin was the culprit agent in a significantly higher percentage of patients with preexisting liver disease compared with those without (6.7% vs 1.5%; $P = .004$), which could potentially be caused by increased use of azithromycin in patients with CLD because of the presumed safety profile of the medication.[16]

Some drugs or classes of drugs are inappropriately avoided, specifically acetaminophen and statins, based on misconceptions. In patients with chronic alcohol intake, there is an increased risk of hepatic coma and death with acetaminophen overdose compared with patients without chronic alcohol intake (relative risk 5.3 vs 1.4, respectively).[37] When acetaminophen is used according to the prescribing label, it is safe. Acetaminophen is considered first-line treatment of pain in patients with cirrhosis and is preferred to nonsteroidal antiinflammatory drugs (NSAIDs) because of the potential for renal dysfunction and gastrointestinal bleeding with NSAID use.[38] Adult patients with cirrhosis should limit acetaminophen doses to no more than 2 g in a 24-hour period. Hepatoxicity of statin therapy has long been a concern among prescribers, although significant increases in liver enzyme levels are rare and do not differ from recipients receiving placebo in large clinic trials.[39,40] The concern for hepatotoxicity has led to hesitation of statin use among patients with CLD. Multiple studies have shown statins can be used safely in patients with and without CLD.[39–43] Changes in liver enzyme levels observed in patients on statins with CLD are more likely to reflect fluctuations in underlying liver disease than any association with statin hepatoxicity.[41] Safety of statin use has been shown in several categories of CLD, including primary biliary cholangitis, hepatitis C virus (HCV), and NAFLD.[44–49] In addition, statins provide important cardiovascular benefits and decrease risk for decompensation, mortality, and hepatocellular carcinoma in patients with cirrhosis.[50–52] Therefore, statins should not be withheld from patients based on underlying liver disease if otherwise clinically indicated. When prescribing potentially hepatotoxic medications to patients with cirrhosis, checking liver chemistries at monthly intervals for 3 months is recommended.[3]

Medications not generally associated with DILI in the healthy population may have the potential for hepatotoxicity in the setting of advanced liver disease. Drugs and classes of drugs that have been shown to have higher risk of hepatotoxicity in patients with underlying liver disease are shown in **Box 2**, and the more commonly used medications are discussed in detail later.[36]

Antiretroviral Therapy for Human Immunodeficiency Virus

Antiretroviral therapy (ART) for HIV can cause liver injury via multiple mechanisms, including hypersensitivity reactions, mitochondrial toxicity, steatosis, and direct liver cell stress.[53] Case reports have been published of patients being treated for HIV developing portal hypertension in the absence of other forms of CLD.[54,55] Both nucleoside reverse transcriptase inhibitors and nonnucleoside reverse transcriptase inhibitors (NNRTIs) can cause hepatotoxicity. Patients with chronic hepatitis B or C receiving NNRTIs had a 2-fold higher risk for severe hepatotoxicity, in some cases requiring transplant or leading to death.[20] NNRTIs should be avoided in patients with Child-Pugh B or C cirrhosis.[53]

The second major issue in treating patients with HIV is differentiating between DILI and reactivation of their hepatitis B virus (HBV) infection. Immune

---

Box 2
Drugs or classes of drugs with suspected or increased risk of hepatotoxicity in chronic liver disease

Antiretroviral therapy

Protease inhibitors

Antituberculosis drugs (isoniazid, pyrazinamide, rifampin)

Obeticholic acid

Methimazole

Methotrexate

Nefazodone

Valproate

Vitamin A

Tamoxifen

reconstitution after starting ART in HIV-HBV coinfection can be challenging to differentiate from DILI. However, these agents are being used less in favor of tenofovir-containing regimens.[20,53] Regimens used to treat HIV in patients with HBV are recommended to include agents with anti-HBV , such as tenofovir, emtricitabine, and lamuvidine.[53] The importance of adherence to ART should be emphasized in patients with HIV and HBV because changes or discontinuation of HBV treatment in this setting can lead to significant worsening of hepatitis and even hepatic failure.[56–60]

Protease Inhibitors

Previous interferon-based regimens for treatment of HCV in patients with decompensated cirrhosis were limited by poor response to treatment, tolerability, and risk of worsening hepatic dysfunction.[61] However, current interferon-free direct-acting antivirals have shown good response in treatment of hepatitis C. However, the transition period between using interferon, ribavirin, and the first-generation protease inhibitors, boceprevir and telaprevir, in patients with hepatitis C–induced cirrhosis was associated with significant hepatic decompensation and death.[62] A second-generation protease inhibitor, simeprevir, was commonly associated with hyperbilirubinemia when used in combination with sofosbuvir and ribavirin.[63] In addition, case reports of patients with hepatitis C–induced cirrhosis treated with protease inhibitors and sofosbuvir have cautioned that the risk of further hepatic decompensation is high in patients with decompensated cirrhosis.[64–70] Thus the American Association for the Study of Liver Diseases and the Infectious Diseases Society of America recommend for those patients with decompensated cirrhosis that the use of protease inhibitor–containing regimens should be done with extreme caution because of potential toxicity.[71] Fortunately, there are other direct-acting antiviral regimens that do not include a protease inhibitor, and these agents have shown benefit in clearing hepatitis C in decompensated cirrhotic patients, without worsening decompensation.[72–75] All patients with decompensated cirrhosis must be monitored closely during HCV treatment and consultation with a liver transplant center is strongly recommended.

Antituberculosis Drugs

Incidence of DILI in patients receiving antituberculosis treatment ranges from 2% to 28%[76–81] with significant mortality. A single-center study reviewing consecutive cases of tuberculosis treatment identified 269 cases (25.7%) with DILI.[82] Of those, 75% occurred within the first 2 months of treatment with a mortality of 22.7% at 90 days. The presence of jaundice, encephalopathy, or ascites was associated with mortalities of 30%, 69.6%, and 50.7%, respectively. Age, gender, transaminase levels, HIV, or hepatitis B surface antigen status did not influence survival.

Risk factors suspected to increase the risk of hepatotoxicity of antituberculosis agents include advanced age (>50 years old), CLD, abuse of alcohol or other drugs, or malnutrition (body mass index <18.5 kg/m^2).[83] Using these risk factors to define a high-risk group, a prospective cohort study showed that the incidence of hepatotoxicity in patients treated with isoniazid, rifampin, and pyrazinamide was 18.2% compared with only 5.8% in patients without these risk factors.[84] The risk of severe hepatotoxicity, defined as an increase of serum transaminase level greater than 10 times the upper limits of normal, was 6.9% versus 0.4% in the high-risk versus low-risk groups, respectively ($P<.001$). Chronic hepatitis C with or without chronic hepatitis B infection may also be a risk factor for DILI in patients receiving tuberculosis treatment.[85–88] When DILI is encountered, antituberculosis treatment agents should be stopped until hepatotoxicity resolves.[89]

Obeticholic Acid

Obeticholic acid (OCA) is a farnesoid X nuclear receptor agonist approved by the FDA in May 2016 to treat adult patients with primary biliary cholangitis. OCA was approved for use in combination with ursodeoxycholic acid (UDCA) in adults with an inadequate response to UDCA, or as monotherapy in adults unable to tolerate UDCA. In the clinical phase 2 and 3 trials, which enrolled 375 patients, there were no safety issues regarding serious liver injury or failure.[90,91] Both trials excluded patients with decompensated cirrhosis (Child-Pugh class B or C).

However, 13 months after FDA approval, the FDA's Adverse Event Reporting System received 19 cases of death. Seven of these cases were attributed to ACLF related to drug hepatotoxicity.[92] The mechanism of injury is not known. In all but 1 of the 7 cases, patients were prescribed doses higher than published recommendations. Manufacturer labeling recommends a starting dose of 5 mg weekly and no more than 10 mg twice weekly for patients with Child-Pugh class B or C cirrhosis. Any increase in liver tests with accompanying hepatic decompensation should lead to immediate discontinuation of OCA.[93]

Rifampin

Rifampin is a semisynthetic antibiotic used to treat bacterial infections, most notably tuberculosis. It was also discovered to aid in pruritus associated with cholestatic liver disease by inducing many of the major cytochrome P450 pathways in the liver and is included in most treatment guidelines.[94–97] DILI caused by rifampin was first described in a case series in 1974.[98] Since then, most instances from rifampin-induced liver injury have been documented in the setting of high dosages of rifampin (600 mg daily), with other tuberculosis treatment agents also known to cause hepatotoxicity, such as isoniazid.[99,100]

Limited safety data are available using rifampin in chronic cholestatic liver diseases for pruritus. A meta-analysis of prospective, randomized-controlled trials using rifampin for the treatment of pruritus caused by chronic cholestasis was only able to identify 5 studies including a total of 61 patients. None of the patients receiving rifampin developed hepatotoxicity; thus, the meta-analysis concluded rifampin for short duration is associated with a low risk of hepatotoxicity.[101] A retrospective study of 105 chronic cholestatic patients treated with rifampin found that 5% of patients developed hepatotoxicity, and all cases resolved with cessation of the rifampin.[102] Thus, based on limited studies and the concern for hepatotoxicity with rifampin, expert opinion recommends to avoid use in the setting of bilirubin level greater than 2.5 mg/dL and to monitor patients closely, especially in the first few months of therapy.[94,103] The recommended starting dose is 150 mg daily with dose titration as needed to a maximum daily dose of 600 mg. In addition, because rifampin induces many of the cytochrome P450 pathways along with the P-glycoprotein pathway, a review of all other medications should be conducted before initiating rifampin for treatment of pruritus in patients with cholestasis.[104]

MANAGEMENT

The most important part of managing patients with DILI in CLD is to quickly identify and discontinue the offending medication. Patients should be counseled on the risk of reexposure and readministration should be avoided.[7,13,105] Management remains largely supportive, although the identification of jaundice or decompensated cirrhosis should prompt consultation with a liver transplant center. Among pharmacologic therapy, options are limited and similar to those in patients without underlying CLD. In cases of suspected or known acetaminophen overdose in patients with CLD, N-acetylcysteine (NAC) remains essential first-line therapy and should be continued until resolution of encephalopathy or INR less than 1.5, as in patients without CLD.[106] Corticosteroids have a role in drug-induced autoimmune hepatitis. Medications and classes of medications that can cause autoimmune hepatitis include nitrofurantoin, hydralazine, methyldopa, fenofibrate, statins, alfa and beta interferons, and tumor necrosis factor inhibitors.[107] There are currently no recommendations to avoid use of these agents in patients with CLD. Commonly used cancer therapies, including tyrosine kinase inhibitors and immune checkpoint inhibitors, also have a risk of causing autoimmune hepatitis. These therapies were not studied in patients with CLD and should likely be avoided in patients with advanced fibrosis or cirrhosis. These patients generally respond to withdrawal of therapy and corticosteroid treatment.[108–110]

PROGNOSIS

Patients with who develop DILI with underlying CLD are at higher risk for poor outcomes.[18,111] In patients without CLD, cholestatic DILI carries better prognosis compared with hepatocellular injury.[3,8] In large population-based studies, hepatocellular injury most often led to liver transplant (3%–6%) or mortality (7%–12%), compared with cholestatic or mixed injury.[2,14,16] However, cholestatic injury is more likely to lead to chronic (>6 months) liver injury (31%), compared with hepatocellular (13%) or mixed (14%) injury in patients both with and without CLD.[16] Hy's law, which predicts at least 10% mortality in patients with DILI who have both hepatocellular injury and jaundice, showed similar outcomes between patients with and without CLD.[16,112–114] The Model for End-stage Liver Disease (MELD) has been identified as an independent predictor of mortality in patients with DILI, but no data are available in the setting of CLD.[115,116]

For patients who develop ACLF from DILI, the prognosis is poor. ACLF refers to acute decompensation of CLD and is associated with organ failure and high short-term mortality.[117–121] ACLF can arise from a variety of insults, with the most common identifiable triggers being bacterial infection, exacerbation of hepatitis B, active alcoholism, and gastrointestinal hemorrhage.[122] DILI as a precipitant for ACLF has been discussed less commonly, but likely plays a significant role. Models predicting mortality for patients with ACLF are available, from the North American Consortium for the Study of End-Stage Liver Disease (NACSELD)[123] and the Chronic Liver Failure Consortium (CLIF-C),[121] affiliated with the European Association for the Study of the Liver, but their role in predicting mortality in patients with DILI and CLD is limited by small numbers of patients.[118,124] The largest database enrolling patients with DILI causing ACLF is the Asian Pacific Association of Study of Liver ACLF Research Consortium (AARC), which examined 3132 patients with ACLF and found that 329 (10.5%) were caused by DILI.[125] Patients with decompensated cirrhosis were excluded from the study. Of the medications implicated, complementary and alternative medicines made up 71.7% of cases, followed by antituberculosis therapy (27.3%), methotrexate (0.6%), and antiepileptics (0.3%). A significantly higher percentage of cases occurred in women versus men (52.3% vs 28.5%; P<.001). Mortality was higher among patients with ACLF caused by DILI than other causes (46.5% vs 38.8%; P = .007), with fatal cases most often attributed to complementary and alternative medicines or antituberculosis therapy. Predictors of 90-day mortality included increased serum creatinine level, total bilirubin, INR, lactate level, and development of hepatic encephalopathy. The cause of CLD was not associated with mortality; however, patients with

DILI-induced ACLF were more likely to have cryptogenic cirrhosis (72% vs 43%; P<.001) and less likely to have alcoholic liver disease (28% vs 56%; P<.001). The European Association for the Study of the Liver–Chronic Liver Failure Consortium (EASL-CLIF) evaluated 303 patients with ACLF.[121] No cases were attributed to DILI; however, 126 (43.6%) did not have an attributable cause. The DILIN did not specifically define or comment on the presence of ACLF; however, they also noted a significantly higher mortality in patients with underlying CLD compared with patients without underlying CLD (16% vs 5.2%; P<.0001).[16]

SUMMARY

DILI in the setting of CLD remains challenging to many practitioners. Although still small in numbers of patients with CLD, large-prospective studies such as the DILIN Prospective Study are increasing the understanding of DILI in CLD. Risk factors for DILI are difficult to assess given its low incidence, but recent studies suggest patients with NAFLD may be more susceptible to DILI, challenging the previous consensus that CLD was not a risk factor for DILI. Presenting clinical features of patients with CLD experiencing DILI are similar to those without CLD, although diabetes is more commonly found in patients with CLD. Classes of offending agents for DILI in CLD are the same as those without CLD, although azithromycin was more commonly seen in patients with CLD. Without reliable biomarkers or assessment tools, diagnosis of DILI in CLD requires a high index of suspicion as well as good clinical judgment given the difficulty in differentiating exacerbations of CLD from drug-induced hepatotoxicity. Early consultation to a liver transplant center should be pursued given evidence of worse outcomes when DILI occurs among patients with CLD.

Caution must be taken when prescribing medicines to patients with underlying liver disease, and the risks versus benefits as well as potential for increased hepatotoxicity among patients with impaired liver function should be considered. Certain medications, such as protease inhibitors, obeticholic acid, rifampin, and some HIV and anti-tuberculosis medications, have concerning hepatotoxicity in some forms of CLD and use should be avoided or closely monitored. LiverTox and MEDWATCH are useful tools for reporting and understanding hepatotoxicity of medications, particularly given the low incidence of DILI and exclusion of patients with CLD from clinical drug development trials. CLD is not a risk factor for statin-induced hepatotoxicity, and, in the appropriate clinical setting, statins can and should be used to improve outcomes in patients with underlying liver disease.

Future research in genomics and personalized medicine will be helpful in identifying and mitigating the risk of DILI in subpopulations, including those with CLD.[4] Discovery of a reliable biomarker will aid in a more precise and reproducible diagnosis of DILI, which continues to be a challenge. Although large, prospective registries, such as the DILIN Prospective Study, will increase the understanding of common CLDs and DILI, the role of less common liver diseases, such as autoimmune hepatitis, in DILI remains understudied.

REFERENCES

1. Sgro C, Clinard F, Ouazir K, et al. Incidence of drug-induced hepatic injuries: a French population-based study. Hepatology 2002;36(2):451–5.
2. Bjornsson ES, Bergmann OM, Bjornsson HK, et al. Incidence, presentation, and outcomes in patients with drug-induced liver injury in the general population of Iceland. Gastroenterology 2013;144(7):1419–25, 1425.e1-3. [quiz: e1419–20].

3. Chalasani NP, Hayashi PH, Bonkovsky HL, et al. ACG Clinical Guideline: the diagnosis and management of idiosyncratic drug-induced liver injury. Am J Gastroenterol 2014;109(7):950–66 [quiz: 967].
4. Lucado J, Paez K, Elixhauser A. Medication-related adverse outcomes in U.S. Hospitals and Emergency Departments, 2008: statistical Brief #109. Healthcare Cost and Utilization Project (HCUP) statistical Briefs. Rockville (MD): Agency for Healthcare Research and Quality (US); 2006.
5. Vuppalanchi R, Liangpunsakul S, Chalasani N. Etiology of new-onset jaundice: how often is it caused by idiosyncratic drug-induced liver injury in the United States? Am J Gastroenterol 2007;102(3):558–62 [quiz: 693].
6. Chalasani N, Fontana RJ, Bonkovsky HL, et al. Causes, clinical features, and outcomes from a prospective study of drug-induced liver injury in the United States. Gastroenterology 2008;135(6):1924–34, 1934.e1-4.
7. Navarro VJ, Senior JR. Drug-related hepatotoxicity. N Engl J Med 2006;354(7): 731–9.
8. Uetrecht J, Naisbitt DJ. Idiosyncratic adverse drug reactions: current concepts. Pharmacol Rev 2013;65(2):779–808.
9. Uetrecht J. Idiosyncratic drug reactions: current understanding. Annu Rev Pharmacol Toxicol 2007;47:513–39.
10. Watkins PB, Seeff LB. Drug-induced liver injury: summary of a single topic clinical research conference. Hepatology 2006;43(3):618–31.
11. Aithal GP, Watkins PB, Andrade RJ, et al. Case definition and phenotype standardization in drug-induced liver injury. Clin Pharmacol Ther 2011;89(6):806–15.
12. Benichou C. Criteria of drug-induced liver disorders. Report of an international consensus meeting. J Hepatol 1990;11(2):272–6.
13. Fontana RJ, Watkins PB, Bonkovsky HL, et al. Drug-Induced Liver Injury Network (DILIN) prospective study: rationale, design and conduct. Drug Saf 2009;32(1):55–68.
14. Andrade RJ, Lucena MI, Fernandez MC, et al. Drug-induced liver injury: an analysis of 461 incidences submitted to the Spanish registry over a 10-year period. Gastroenterology 2005;129(2):512–21.
15. De Valle MB, Av Klinteberg V, Alem N, et al. Drug-induced liver injury in a Swedish University hospital out-patient hepatology clinic. Aliment Pharmacol Ther 2006;24(8):1187–95.
16. Chalasani N, Bonkovsky HL, Fontana R, et al. Features and outcomes of 899 patients with drug-induced liver injury: the DILIN prospective study. Gastroenterology 2015;148(7):1340–52.e7.
17. Younossi Z, Anstee QM, Marietti M, et al. Global burden of NAFLD and NASH: trends, predictions, risk factors and prevention. Nat Rev Gastroenterol Hepatol 2018;15(1):11–20.
18. Zimmerman H. Hepatotoxicity: the adverse effects of drugs and other chemicals on the liver. 2nd edition. Philadelphia: Lippincott Williams & Wilkins; 1999.
19. Lammert C, Einarsson S, Saha C, et al. Relationship between daily dose of oral medications and idiosyncratic drug-induced liver injury: search for signals. Hepatology 2008;47(6):2003–9.
20. Sulkowski MS, Thomas DL, Chaisson RE, et al. Hepatotoxicity associated with antiretroviral therapy in adults infected with human immunodeficiency virus and the role of hepatitis C or B virus infection. JAMA 2000;283(1):74–80.
21. Wong WM, Wu PC, Yuen MF, et al. Antituberculosis drug-related liver dysfunction in chronic hepatitis B infection. Hepatology 2000;31(1):201–6.

22. Ungo JR, Jones D, Ashkin D, et al. Antituberculosis drug-induced hepatotoxic-
    ity. The role of hepatitis C virus and the human immunodeficiency virus. Am J
    Respir Crit Care Med 1998;157(6 Pt 1):1871–6.
23. Russo MW, Watkins PB. Are patients with elevated liver tests at increased risk of
    drug-induced liver injury? Gastroenterology 2004;126(5):1477–80.
24. Tarantino G, Conca P, Basile V, et al. A prospective study of acute drug-induced
    liver injury in patients suffering from non-alcoholic fatty liver disease. Hepatol
    Res 2007;37(6):410–5.
25. Lammert C, Imler T, Teal E, et al. Patients with chronic liver disease suggestive
    of nonalcoholic fatty liver disease may Be at higher risk for drug-induced liver
    injury. Clin Gastroenterol Hepatol 2018. [Epub ahead of print].
26. Kaplowitz N. Causality assessment versus guilt-by-association in drug hepato-
    toxicity. Hepatology 2001;33(1):308–10.
27. Rockey DC, Seeff LB, Rochon J, et al. Causality assessment in drug-induced
    liver injury using a structured expert opinion process: comparison to the
    Roussel-Uclaf causality assessment method. Hepatology 2010;51(6):2117–26.
28. Agarwal VK, McHutchison JG, Hoofnagle JH. Drug-Induced Liver Injury N.
    Important elements for the diagnosis of drug-induced liver injury. Clin Gastroen-
    terol Hepatol 2010;8(5):463–70.
29. Danan G, Benichou C. Causality assessment of adverse reactions to drugs–I. A
    novel method based on the conclusions of international consensus meetings:
    application to drug-induced liver injuries. J Clin Epidemiol 1993;46(11):
    1323–30.
30. Benichou C, Danan G, Flahault A. Causality assessment of adverse reactions to
    drugs–II. An original model for validation of drug causality assessment methods:
    case reports with positive rechallenge. J Clin Epidemiol 1993;46(11):1331–6.
31. Teschke R, Andrade RJ. Drug-induced liver injury: expanding our knowledge by
    enlarging population analysis with prospective and scoring causality assess-
    ment. Gastroenterology 2015;148(7):1271–3.
32. Rochon J, Protiva P, Seeff LB, et al. Reliability of the Roussel Uclaf causality
    assessment method for assessing causality in drug-induced liver injury. Hepa-
    tology 2008;48(4):1175–83.
33. Maria VA, Victorino RM. Development and validation of a clinical scale for the
    diagnosis of drug-induced hepatitis. Hepatology 1997;26(3):664–9.
34. LiverTox. Available at: https://livertox.nih.gov. Accessed May 11, 2019.
35. Watkins PB. Idiosyncratic liver injury: challenges and approaches. Toxicol
    Pathol 2005;33(1):1–5.
36. Lewis JH, Stine JG. Review article: prescribing medications in patients with
    cirrhosis - a practical guide. Aliment Pharmacol Ther 2013;37(12):1132–56.
37. Schiodt FV, Lee WM, Bondesen S, et al. Influence of acute and chronic alcohol
    intake on the clinical course and outcome in acetaminophen overdose. Aliment
    Pharmacol Ther 2002;16(4):707–15.
38. Chandok N, Watt KD. Pain management in the cirrhotic patient: the clinical chal-
    lenge. Mayo Clin Proc 2010;85(5):451–8.
39. de Denus S, Spinler SA, Miller K, et al. Statins and liver toxicity: a meta-analysis.
    Pharmacotherapy 2004;24(5):584–91.
40. Pfeffer MA, Keech A, Sacks FM, et al. Safety and tolerability of pravastatin in
    long-term clinical trials: prospective Pravastatin Pooling (PPP) Project. Circula-
    tion 2002;105(20):2341–6.

41. Chalasani N, Aljadhey H, Kesterson J, et al. Patients with elevated liver enzymes are not at higher risk for statin hepatotoxicity. Gastroenterology 2004;126(5): 1287–92.

42. Vuppalanchi R, Teal E, Chalasani N. Patients with elevated baseline liver enzymes do not have higher frequency of hepatotoxicity from lovastatin than those with normal baseline liver enzymes. Am J Med Sci 2005;329(2):62–5.

43. Lewis JH, Mortensen ME, Zweig S, et al. Efficacy and safety of high-dose pravastatin in hypercholesterolemic patients with well-compensated chronic liver disease: results of a prospective, randomized, double-blind, placebo-controlled, multicenter trial. Hepatology 2007;46(5):1453–63.

44. Kurihara T, Akimoto M, Abe K, et al. Experimental use of pravastatin in patients with primary biliary cirrhosis associated with hypercholesterolemia. Clin Ther 1993;15(5):890–8.

45. Ritzel U, Leonhardt U, Nather M, et al. Simvastatin in primary biliary cirrhosis: effects on serum lipids and distinct disease markers. J Hepatol 2002;36(4):454–8.

46. Khorashadi S, Hasson NK, Cheung RC. Incidence of statin hepatotoxicity in patients with hepatitis C. Clin Gastroenterol Hepatol 2006;4(7):902–7 [quiz: 806].

47. Gibson K, Rindone JP. Experience with statin use in patients with chronic hepatitis C infection. Am J Cardiol 2005;96(9):1278–9.

48. Cohen DE, Anania FA, Chalasani N. National lipid association statin safety task force liver expert P. An assessment of statin safety by hepatologists. Am J Cardiol 2006;97(8A):77C–81C.

49. Rallidis LS, Drakoulis CK, Parasi AS. Pravastatin in patients with nonalcoholic steatohepatitis: results of a pilot study. Atherosclerosis 2004;174(1):193–6.

50. Chang FM, Wang YP, Lang HC, et al. Statins decrease the risk of decompensation in hepatitis B virus- and hepatitis C virus-related cirrhosis: a population-based study. Hepatology 2017;66(3):896–907.

51. Butt AA, Yan P, Bonilla H, et al. Effect of addition of statins to antiviral therapy in hepatitis C virus-infected persons: results from ERCHIVES. Hepatology 2015; 62(2):365–74.

52. Athyros VG, Tziomalos K, Gossios TD, et al. Safety and efficacy of long-term statin treatment for cardiovascular events in patients with coronary heart disease and abnormal liver tests in the Greek Atorvastatin and Coronary Heart Disease Evaluation (GREACE) Study: a post-hoc analysis. Lancet 2010;376(9756): 1916–22.

53. Nunez M. Clinical syndromes and consequences of antiretroviral-related hepatotoxicity. Hepatology 2010;52(3):1143–55.

54. Maida I, Nunez M, Rios MJ, et al. Severe liver disease associated with prolonged exposure to antiretroviral drugs. J Acquir Immune Defic Syndr 2006; 42(2):177–82.

55. Maida I, Garcia-Gasco P, Sotgiu G, et al. Antiretroviral-associated portal hypertension: a new clinical condition? Prevalence, predictors and outcome. Antivir Ther 2008;13(1):103–7.

56. Bessesen M, Ives D, Condreay L, et al. Chronic active hepatitis B exacerbations in human immunodeficiency virus-infected patients following development of resistance to or withdrawal of lamivudine. Clin Infect Dis 1999;28(5):1032–5.

57. Altfeld M, Rockstroh JK, Addo M, et al. Reactivation of hepatitis B in a long-term anti-HBs-positive patient with AIDS following lamivudine withdrawal. J Hepatol 1998;29(2):306–9.

58. McGovern B. What drives hepatitis B virus-related hepatic flares? Virus, T cells–or a bit of both? Clin Infect Dis 2004;39(1):133–5.

59. Dore GJ, Soriano V, Rockstroh J, et al. Frequent hepatitis B virus rebound among HIV-hepatitis B virus-coinfected patients following antiretroviral therapy interruption. AIDS 2010;24(6):857–65.
60. Bellini C, Keiser O, Chave JP, et al. Liver enzyme elevation after lamivudine withdrawal in HIV-hepatitis B virus co-infected patients: the Swiss HIV Cohort Study. HIV Med 2009;10(1):12–8.
61. Banerjee D, Reddy KR. Review article: safety and tolerability of direct-acting anti-viral agents in the new era of hepatitis C therapy. Aliment Pharmacol Ther 2016;43(6):674–96.
62. Hezode C, Fontaine H, Dorival C, et al. Effectiveness of telaprevir or boceprevir in treatment-experienced patients with HCV genotype 1 infection and cirrhosis. Gastroenterology 2014;147(1):132–42.e4.
63. Lawitz E, Sulkowski MS, Ghalib R, et al. Simeprevir plus sofosbuvir, with or without ribavirin, to treat chronic infection with hepatitis C virus genotype 1 in non-responders to pegylated interferon and ribavirin and treatment-naive patients: the COSMOS randomised study. Lancet 2014;384(9956):1756–65.
64. Stine JG, Intagliata N, Shah NL, et al. Hepatic decompensation likely attributable to simeprevir in patients with advanced cirrhosis. Dig Dis Sci 2015;60(4):1031–5.
65. Saxena V, Nyberg L, Pauly M, et al. Safety and efficacy of simeprevir/sofosbuvir in hepatitis C-infected patients with compensated and decompensated cirrhosis. Hepatology 2015;62(3):715–25.
66. Sulkowski MS, Vargas HE, Di Bisceglie AM, et al. Effectiveness of simeprevir plus sofosbuvir, with or without ribavirin, in real-world patients with HCV genotype 1 infection. Gastroenterology 2016;150(2):419–29.
67. Hoofnagle JH. Hepatic decompensation during direct-acting antiviral therapy of chronic hepatitis C. J Hepatol 2016;64(4):763–5.
68. Masetti M, Magalotti D, Martino E, et al. A case of acute liver failure during ritonavir-boosted paritaprevir, ombitasvir and dasabuvir therapy in a patient with HCV genotype 1b cirrhosis. J Gastrointestin Liver Dis 2016;25(4):559–61.
69. Buzas C, Tantau M, Ciobanu L. Fatal acute liver failure during ritonavir-boosted paritaprevir, ombitasvir and dasabuvir plus ribavirin therapy. J Gastrointestin Liver Dis 2017;26(1):93–4.
70. Zeuzem S, Ghalib R, Reddy KR, et al. Grazoprevir-elbasvir combination therapy for treatment-naive cirrhotic and noncirrhotic patients with chronic hepatitis C virus genotype 1, 4, or 6 infection: a randomized trial. Ann Intern Med 2015;163(1):1–13.
71. Panel A-IHG. Hepatitis C guidance 2018 update: AASLD-IDSA recommendations for testing, managing, and treating hepatitis C virus infection. Clin Infect Dis 2018;67(10):1477–92.
72. Manns M, Samuel D, Gane EJ, et al. Ledipasvir and sofosbuvir plus ribavirin in patients with genotype 1 or 4 hepatitis C virus infection and advanced liver disease: a multicentre, open-label, randomised, phase 2 trial. Lancet Infect Dis 2016;16(6):685–97.
73. Curry MP, O'Leary JG, Bzowej N, et al. Sofosbuvir and Velpatasvir for HCV in patients with decompensated cirrhosis. N Engl J Med 2015;373(27):2618–28.
74. Charlton M, Everson GT, Flamm SL, et al. Ledipasvir and sofosbuvir plus ribavirin for treatment of HCV infection in patients with advanced liver disease. Gastroenterology 2015;149(3):649–59.
75. Welzel TM, Petersen J, Herzer K, et al. Daclatasvir plus sofosbuvir, with or without ribavirin, achieved high sustained virological response rates in patients with HCV

infection and advanced liver disease in a real-world cohort. Gut 2016;65(11): 1861–70.

76. Sharifzadeh M, Rasoulinejad M, Valipour F, et al. Evaluation of patient-related factors associated with causality, preventability, predictability and severity of hepatotoxicity during antituberculosis [correction of antituberclosis] treatment. Pharmacol Res 2005;51(4):353–8.

77. Sharma SK, Balamurugan A, Saha PK, et al. Evaluation of clinical and immuno-genetic risk factors for the development of hepatotoxicity during antituberculosis treatment. Am J Respir Crit Care Med 2002;166(7):916–9.

78. van Hest R, Baars H, Kik S, et al. Hepatotoxicity of rifampin-pyrazinamide and isoniazid preventive therapy and tuberculosis treatment. Clin Infect Dis 2004; 39(4):488–96.

79. Tost JR, Vidal R, Cayla J, et al. Severe hepatotoxicity due to anti-tuberculosis drugs in Spain. Int J Tuberc Lung Dis 2005;9(5):534–40.

80. Singanayagam A, Sridhar S, Dhariwal J, et al. A comparison between two strategies for monitoring hepatic function during antituberculous therapy. Am J Respir Crit Care Med 2012;185(6):653–9.

81. Blumberg HM, Burman WJ, Chaisson RE, et al. American Thoracic Society/Centers for Disease Control and Prevention/Infectious Diseases Society of America: treatment of tuberculosis. Am J Respir Crit Care Med 2003;167(4):603–62.

82. Devarbhavi H, Singh R, Patil M, et al. Outcome and determinants of mortality in 269 patients with combination anti-tuberculosis drug-induced liver injury. J Gastroenterol Hepatol 2013;28(1):161–7.

83. Makhlouf HA, Helmy A, Fawzy E, et al. A prospective study of antituberculous drug-induced hepatotoxicity in an area endemic for liver diseases. Hepatol Int 2008;2(3):353–60.

84. Fernandez-Villar A, Sopena B, Fernandez-Villar J, et al. The influence of risk factors on the severity of anti-tuberculosis drug-induced hepatotoxicity. Int J Tuberc Lung Dis 2004;8(12):1499–505.

85. Lomtadze N, Kupreishvili L, Salakaia A, et al. Hepatitis C virus co-infection increases the risk of anti-tuberculosis drug-induced hepatotoxicity among patients with pulmonary tuberculosis. PLoS One 2013;8(12):e83892.

86. Fernandez-Villar A, Sopena B, Garcia J, et al. Hepatitis C virus RNA in serum as a risk factor for isoniazid hepatotoxicity. Infection 2007;35(4):295–7.

87. Liu YM, Cheng YJ, Li YL, et al. Antituberculosis treatment and hepatotoxicity in patients with chronic viral hepatitis. Lung 2014;192(1):205–10.

88. Kim WS, Lee SS, Lee CM, et al. Hepatitis C and not Hepatitis B virus is a risk factor for anti-tuberculosis drug induced liver injury. BMC Infect Dis 2016;16:50.

89. Saukkonen JJ, Cohn DL, Jasmer RM, et al. An official ATS statement: hepatotoxicity of antituberculosis therapy. Am J Respir Crit Care Med 2006;174(8):935–52.

90. Hirschfield GM, Mason A, Luketic V, et al. Efficacy of obeticholic acid in patients with primary biliary cirrhosis and inadequate response to ursodeoxycholic acid. Gastroenterology 2015;148(4):751–61.e8.

91. Nevens F, Andreone P, Mazzella G, et al. A placebo-controlled trial of obeticholic acid in primary biliary cholangitis. N Engl J Med 2016;375(7):631–43.

92. Administration FaD. FDA adds Boxed Warning to highlight correct dosing of Ocaliva (obeticholic acid) for patients with a rare chronic liver disease. 2018. Available at: https://www.fda.gov/drugs/drug-safety-and-availability/fda-adds-boxed-warning-highlight-correct-dosing-ocaliva-obeticholic-acid-patients-rare-chronic-liver. Accessed May 11, 2019.

93. Brown RS Jr. Use of obeticholic acid in patients with primary biliary cholangitis. Gastroenterol Hepatol 2018;14(11):654–7.
94. Bachs L, Pares A, Elena M, et al. Comparison of rifampicin with phenobarbitone for treatment of pruritus in biliary cirrhosis. Lancet 1989;1(8638):574–6.
95. Loginov AS, Reshetniak VI, Petrakov AV. The treatment of primary biliary liver cirrhosis with rifampicin. Ter Arkh 1993;65(8):57–62.
96. Podesta A, Lopez P, Terg R, et al. Treatment of pruritus of primary biliary cirrhosis with rifampin. Dig Dis Sci 1991;36(2):216–20.
97. Ghent CN, Carruthers SG. Treatment of pruritus in primary biliary cirrhosis with rifampin. Results of a double-blind, crossover, randomized trial. Gastroenterology 1988;94(2):488–93.
98. Scheuer PJ, Summerfield JA, Lal S, et al. Rifampicin hepatitis. A clinical and histological study. Lancet 1974;1(7855):421–5.
99. Lees AW, Allan GW, Smith J, et al. Toxicity form rifampicin plus isoniazid and rifampicin plus ethambutol therapy. Tubercle 1971;52(3):182–90.
100. Hollins PJ, Simmons AV. Jaundice associated with rifampicin. Tubercle 1970; 51(3):328–32.
101. Khurana S, Singh P. Rifampin is safe for treatment of pruritus due to chronic cholestasis: a meta-analysis of prospective randomized-controlled trials. Liver Int 2006;26(8):943–8.
102. Webb GJ, Rahman SR, Levy C, et al. Low risk of hepatotoxicity from rifampicin when used for cholestatic pruritus: a cross-disease cohort study. Aliment Pharmacol Ther 2018;47(8):1213–9.
103. Prince MI, Burt AD, Jones DE. Hepatitis and liver dysfunction with rifampicin therapy for pruritus in primary biliary cirrhosis. Gut 2002;50(3):436–9.
104. Markowitz JS, DeVane CL. Rifampin-induced selective serotonin reuptake inhibitor withdrawal syndrome in a patient treated with sertraline. J Clin Psychopharmacol 2000;20(1):109–10.
105. Kessler DA. Introducing MEDWatch. A new approach to reporting medication and device adverse effects and product problems. JAMA 1993;269(21):2765–8.
106. Smilkstein MJ, Knapp GL, Kulig KW, et al. Efficacy of oral N-acetylcysteine in the treatment of acetaminophen overdose. Analysis of the national multicenter study (1976 to 1985). N Engl J Med 1988;319(24):1557–62.
107. Autoimmune hepatitis. Available at: https://livertox.nih.gov/Phenotypes_auto. html. Accessed May 12, 2019.
108. Lee T, Lee YS, Yoon SY, et al. Characteristics of liver injury in drug-induced systemic hypersensitivity reactions. J Am Acad Dermatol 2013;69(3):407–15.
109. Puzanov I, Diab A, Abdallah K, et al. Managing toxicities associated with immune checkpoint inhibitors: consensus recommendations from the Society for Immunotherapy of cancer (SITC) toxicity management Working group. J Immunother Cancer 2017;5(1):95.
110. Wang DY, Salem JE, Cohen JV, et al. Fatal toxic effects associated with immune checkpoint inhibitors: a systematic review and meta-analysis. JAMA Oncol 2018;4(12):1721–8.
111. Vuppalanchi R, Chalasani N. Risk factors for drug-induced liver disease. In: Kaplowitz N, Deleve L, editors. Drug-induced liver disease. 3rd edition. London: Academic Press; 2013. p. 265–74.
112. Bjornsson E. Drug-induced liver injury: Hy's rule revisited. Clin Pharmacol Ther 2006;79(6):521–8.
113. Kaplowitz N. Idiosyncratic drug hepatotoxicity. Nat Rev Drug Discov 2005;4(6): 489–99.

114. Bjornsson E, Olsson R. Suspected drug-induced liver fatalities reported to the WHO database. Digestive Liver Dis 2006;38(1):33–8.
115. Rathi C, Pipaliya N, Patel R, et al. Drug induced liver injury at a tertiary hospital in India: etiology, clinical features and predictors of mortality. Ann Hepatol 2017; 16(3):442–50.
116. Devarbhavi H, Patil M, Reddy VV, et al. Drug-induced acute liver failure in children and adults: results of a single-centre study of 128 patients. Liver Int 2018; 38(7):1322–9.
117. Sarin SK, Kumar A, Almeida JA, et al. Acute-on-chronic liver failure: consensus recommendations of the Asian Pacific Association for the study of the liver (APASL). Hepatol Int 2009;3(1):269–82.
118. Sarin SK, Kedarisetty CK, Abbas Z, et al. Acute-on-chronic liver failure: consensus recommendations of the Asian Pacific association for the study of the liver (APASL) 2014. Hepatol Int 2014;8(4):453–71.
119. Bajaj JS, O'Leary JG, Reddy KR, et al. Survival in infection-related acute-on-chronic liver failure is defined by extrahepatic organ failures. Hepatology 2014;60(1):250–6.
120. Jalan R, Yurdaydin C, Bajaj JS, et al. Toward an improved definition of acute-on-chronic liver failure. Gastroenterology 2014;147(1):4–10.
121. Moreau R, Jalan R, Gines P, et al. Acute-on-chronic liver failure is a distinct syndrome that develops in patients with acute decompensation of cirrhosis. Gastroenterology 2013;144(7):1426–37, 1437.e1-9.
122. Hernaez R, Sola E, Moreau R, et al. Acute-on-chronic liver failure: an update. Gut 2017;66(3):541–53.
123. O'Leary JG, Reddy KR, Garcia-Tsao G, et al. NACSELD acute-on-chronic liver failure (NACSELD-ACLF) score predicts 30-day survival in hospitalized patients with cirrhosis. Hepatology 2018;67(6):2367–74.
124. Jalan R, Saliba F, Pavesi M, et al. Development and validation of a prognostic score to predict mortality in patients with acute-on-chronic liver failure. J Hepatol 2014;61(5):1038–47.
125. Devarbhavi H, Choudhury AK, Sharma MK, et al. Drug-induced acute-on-chronic liver failure in Asian patients. Am J Gastroenterol 2019;114(6):929–37.

Drug-Induced Liver Injury from Statins

Lindsay Meurer, MD[a], Stanley Martin Cohen, MD[b],*

KEYWORDS

- Drug-induced liver injury (DILI) • Hydroxymethylglutaryl-CoA reductase inhibitors
- Statins • Liver function test • Hepatotoxicity

KEY POINTS

- Hepatotoxicity rarely occurs with statins.
- Concern for hepatotoxicity should not be a reason to avoid the use of statins in patients with appropriate cardiovascular and cerebrovascular clinical indications.
- Liver function should be tested at the initiation of a statin and as clinically indicated while on therapy. Routine monitoring of liver function while on statin therapy is no longer recommended.
- Diagnostic and therapeutic algorithms exist to help guide clinicians in assessing the patient with possible statin-induced liver injury.
- Statins can be safely used in patients with underlying liver disease, but should be avoided in liver failure, acute liver injury, and decompensated cirrhosis.

INTRODUCTION

The hydroxymethyglutaryl-coenzyme A (HMG-CoA) reductase inhibitors (also known as statins) are a very commonly prescribed class of medications for the treatment of hyperlipidemia, coronary artery disease (CAD), and other atherosclerotic diseases. Statins are associated with a decrease in mortality related to CAD. However, there can be side effects seen with this class of medications. In this article, we will summarize the current data on statin-associated hepatotoxicity and idiosyncratic drug-induced liver injury (DILI).

STATINS: MECHANISM OF ACTION, INDICATIONS, AND ADVERSE EFFECTS

Statins are a class of medications that work by inhibiting the enzyme HMG-CoA reductase, a critical rate-limiting step in the biosynthetic pathway of cholesterol. Owing to

[a] Department of Internal Medicine, University Hospitals Cleveland Medical Center, Case Western Reserve University School of Medicine, 11100 Euclid Avenue, Cleveland, OH 44106, USA; [b] University Hospitals Cleveland Medical Center, Case Western Reserve University School of Medicine, Digestive Health Institute, 11100 Euclid Avenue, Cleveland, OH 44106, USA
* Corresponding author.
E-mail address: Stanley.Cohen@UHhospitals.org

Clin Liver Dis 24 (2020) 107–119
https://doi.org/10.1016/j.cld.2019.09.007
1089-3261/20/© 2019 Elsevier Inc. All rights reserved.

liver.theclinics.com

their significant reduction of cholesterol, namely low-density lipoprotein cholesterol, statins are a key treatment in both primary and secondary prevention of CAD and atherosclerotic disease equivalents.[1] Statins are one of the only lipid-lowering agents with a strong body of evidence proving their cardiovascular benefits, including a decrease in all-cause mortality and reduction in cardiovascular events and stroke.[2] Currently available statins include lovastatin, pravastatin, simvastatin, fluvastatin, atorvastatin, rosuvastatin, and pitavastatin. Atorvastatin, lovastatin, simvastatin, and fluvastatin are lipophilic and are metabolized by the cytochrome P-450 system, pravastatin and pitavastatin are hydrophilic and undergo minimal hepatic metabolization, and rosuvastatin has an intermediate behavior.[1] Statins are generally well-tolerated; however, in some cases, the adverse side effects may limit the use of these life-saving medications.[3] The most commonly reported adverse effects include muscular toxicity ranging from myalgias (seen in 1%–15% of cases) to the more serious complication of rhabdomyolysis.[4] Other potential adverse effects include hepatic and renal dysfunction, and a possible increased risk of diabetes.[5]

Statin use may be associated with a slight increase in transaminases. Up to 3% of patients develop mild transaminase elevations within the first year of statin therapy, but these increases are rarely associated with symptoms and often resolve spontaneously, despite continued statin therapy.[4,6,7] A 2003 meta-analysis of current clinical trials involving statins failed to demonstrate a significant increased risk of elevated liver enzymes compared with placebo for low to moderate dose pravastatin, lovastatin, and simvastatin. Fluvastatin was the only drug associated with an increased risk of liver function abnormalities compared with placebo.[8] A comparative safety analysis of 49 complete trials involving atorvastatin revealed that persistent elevation in hepatic transaminases more than 3 times the upper limit of normal (ULN) was rare, only observed in 0.1%, 0.6%, and 0.2% of patients treated with atorvastatin 10 mg, atorvastatin 80 mg, and placebo, respectively.[9] Liver toxicity is felt to be a class effect with the increased risk of elevated liver enzymes with increasing statin dose.[10,11] This isolated increase in aminotransferases in the absence of elevated bilirubin is not clearly linked to clinically or pathologically relevant liver injury. Other proposed mechanisms for this elevation include transient pharmacologic effect owing to cholesterol reduction in hepatocytes, reflection of muscle injury, coexisting nonalcoholic fatty liver disease (NAFLD), or other unidentified causes of liver injury.[12]

CLINICAL PRESENTATION, DIAGNOSIS, AND OUTCOMES OF DRUG-INDUCED LIVER INJURY IN THE SETTING OF STATIN USE

Statin therapy may cause a mild increase in transaminases; however, this rarely represents clinically relevant liver injury. Compounding this problem is the lack of a consensus agreement on what actually constitutes DILI. Several major studies from the United States, Iceland, Sweden, and Spain provide further insight into the burden of DILI from statins (**Table 1**). These studies also attempt to determine the clinical importance and significance of the associated liver injury.

The US Drug-Induced Liver Injury Network (DILIN) is a multicenter prospective study group aiming to evaluate DILI in the United States from 2004 onward. A 2014 DILIN study by Russo and colleagues[6] sought to describe statin DILI. A study population of 1188 patients suspected to have DILI between 2004 and 2012 were identified. Statins were initially implicated in 61 cases (6%). However, after formal review and adjudication, only 22 cases (1.85%) were felt to truly represent statin-induced DILI demonstrating a potential for overrepresentation in other studies without such a strict

Table 1
Epidemiology and Presentation of presumed Statin-Induced DILI

Study	No. of DILI Cases Attributed to Statins	Hepatocellular Pattern	Cholestatic Pattern	Median Initial Value and Range			No. with Chronic Injury at 6 mo
				ALT	ALP	Bilirubin	
US DILIN[6]	22 of 1188 cases of DILI (1.85%)	12 of 22 (54%)	9 of 22 (41%)	892 U/L (73–3074)	338 U/L (79–1952)	3.9 mg/dL (0.3–18)	4 (18.2%)
Iceland Study[13]	3 of 96 cases of DILI (3.1%)	–	–	–	–	–	–
Swedish Study[14]	8 of 747 cases of DILI (1.1%)	–	–	–	–	–	–
Spanish Hepatotoxicity Registry[16]	47 of 858 cases of DILI (5.5%)	24 of 47 (51.1%)	23 of 47 (48.94%)	17× ULN (1.95–90.17)	2.96× ULN (0.51–15.92)	5.3× ULN (0.2–20.4)	9 (19.1%)

adjudication process. Liver injury was largely mild to moderate and self-limited in nature; however, there were 4 cases that were considered severe and 1 that ultimately lead to death. The majority of cases demonstrated a hepatocellular pattern of liver injury (n = 12). Patients with hepatocellular pattern tended to be younger (mean age, 57 vs 65 years), but did not differ by type of statin, distribution of latencies, gender, body mass index, or disease severity. Fifteen patients (68%) were jaundiced (total bilirubin of ≥2.5 mg/dL) and 4 (18%) had elevations in the serum international normalized ratio (>1.5). The implicated statins included atorvastatin (n = 8), simvastatin (n = 5), rosuvastatin (n = 4), fluvastatin (n = 2), pravastatin (n = 2), and lovastatin (n = 1). The latency from time of initial statin exposure to clinically evident DILI varied widely from 34 days to more than 10 years. This case series concluded that DILI from statins is rare (1.85%), mild to moderate in intensity, self-limited, and likely represents a class effect with idiosyncratic timing of onset and variable presentation.

Another prospective study was performed by Björnsson and colleagues[13] in Iceland collecting data on all cases of DILI from 2010 through 2011. Liver injury was defined as an elevation of alanine aminotransferase (ALT) more than 3 times the ULN and/or an increase in alkaline phosphatase (ALP) greater than 2 times the ULN. A total of 96 patients were identified to have DILI. Statin-induced DILI was observed in 3.1% of patients (atorvastatin, n = 2; and simvastatin, n = 1). Based on the number of patients prescribed atorvastatin, the population risk of DILI was estimated to be 27 per 100,000 (95% confidence interval, 4–98) people treated with atorvastatin.

Björnsson and colleagues[14] retrospectively looked at the incidence of statin-induced DILI using the Swedish Adverse Drug Reactions Advisory Committee from 1970 to 2004. They identified that 8 of 747 of all DILI patients (1.1%) (with jaundice) had suspected statin-induced DILI. Björnsson and colleagues[15] also performed another study using the Swedish Adverse Drug Reactions Advisory Committee to further study hepatotoxicity associated with statins from 1988 to 2010. DILI was defined as aminotransferases greater than 5 times the ULN and/or ALP or bilirubin greater than 2 times the ULN. A total of 73 patients were identified with probable statin-induced liver injury from 1988 until 2010. Overall, statin-related DILI was reported in 1.6 per 100,000 person-years and in 1.2 per 100,000 statin users. Once again, the predominant pattern of injury was hepatocellular (n = 43, 59%), 22 (30%) were cholestatic, and 8 (11%) were of mixed phenotype. Atorvastatin was associated with a cholestatic-predominate phenotype. The implicated statins were as follows: atorvastatin (n = 30), simvastatin (n = 28), fluvastatin (n = 11), pravastatin (n = 2), and rosuvastatin (n = 2).

Another study used the Spanish Hepatotoxicity Registry to study the association of statins with DILI.[16] Two successive definitions of DILI were used in this study. The first definition that was used was derived from the international consensus group in 1989, requiring ALT or conjugated bilirubin greater than 2 times the ULN or a combination of aspartate aminotransferase (AST), ALP, or total bilirubin greater than twice the ULN. The second definition was derived from 2011 revised consensus definition of isolated AST or ALT greater than or equal to 5 times the ULN, ALP greater than 2 times the ULN, or combination of ALT greater than 3 times the ULN and total bilirubin greater than 2 times the ULN. Between April 1994 and August 2012, a total of 858 patients with DILI were identified and statins were implicated in 47 cases (5.5%). The predominant pattern of liver injury was hepatocellular (n = 24, 51%). Jaundice was present in 25 patients (53%). The average time to recovery was 153 days with only 9 patients (19%) having chronic liver injury. The distribution by type of statin was 16 atorvastatin (34%), 13 simvastatin (27.7%), 12 fluvastatin (25.5%), 4 lovastatin (8.5%), and 2 pravastatin (4.3%).

As detailed elsewhere in this article, current evidence suggests that most statin associated DILI is self-limited and resolves without leading to chronic liver injury or death. Similar outcomes are seen with other causes of DILI.[17] Hy Zimmerman's law (Hy's law) for predicting serious liver toxicity suggested a 10% mortality risk in DILI cases with the following: (1) AST or ALT more than 3 times the ULN; (2) serum total bilirubin more than 2 times the ULN without elevation of ALP; and (3) no other reason for the increase in transaminases or bilirubin (absence of acute or chronic liver disease).[18] Russo and colleagues[19] used the United Network for Organ Sharing database from 1990 to 2002 to identify individuals in need of liver transplant related to DILI. Of the 270 patients identified, only 1 case was related to statin use (simvastatin).

HISTOLOGY

Liver biopsies are not always indicated in the evaluated of DILI; however, they can be helpful in excluding other causes of liver injury. Histologic data in the setting of statin-induced liver injury are limited.[20] The DILIN study referenced previously, reported histologic findings in those patients in which biopsy specimens were obtained.[6] Four cases were found to have predominant cholestatic hepatitis with bile duct injury combined with portal and lobular inflammation, and 3 had features of autoimmune hepatitis. Six of 22 had prominent autoimmune features as defined by elevated level of autoantibodies (antinuclear antibody or anti-smooth muscle enzyme >1:80) or liver biopsy suggestive of autoimmune hepatitis. Autoimmune features made the chance of chronic liver disease more likely. Steatosis was commonly found in 5 of 8 biopsies, which likely represented preexisting fatty liver disease. A few other case reports have also demonstrated the association of autoimmune hepatitis with statin use.[21,22]

MONITORING FOR STATIN-RELATED DRUG-INDUCED LIVER INJURY

As the previous studies demonstrated, statins are a rare cause of idiosyncratic DILI; therefore, the need for monitoring of liver function studies has been a topic of discussion. Initial US Food and Drug Administration (FDA) package inserts for statin drugs recommended that clinicians check liver enzymes before starting this class of medication, semiannually, and after dose increases.[23] In 2006, the first National Lipid Association Statin Safety Task Force Expert Liver Panel recommended that routine liver enzyme testing is not required in patients receiving long-term statin therapy.[24] The FDA reassessed the data on statin-induced DILI and concluded that serious liver injury with statins is rare and unpredictable in individual patients, and that routine periodic monitoring of liver enzymes does not seem to be effective in detecting or preventing serious liver injury.[25] The FDA cholesterol-lowering medication safety label update in 2012 reflected this, stating that liver enzymes should be tested before the initiation of statin therapy and only as clinically indicated thereafter. Routine periodic monitoring of liver enzymes in asymptomatic patients taking statins was no longer recommended. The 2014 update by the Statin Liver Safety Task Force supported this monitoring strategy.[26]

DIAGNOSTIC AND THERAPEUTIC APPROACH TO STATIN-RELATED DRUG-INDUCED LIVER INJURY

The 2014 Statin Liver Safety Task Force has developed a comprehensive decision-making tool to assist clinicians in approaching elevation of liver enzymes when considering starting a statin or development of liver test elevation in the setting of on-going statin use (**Figs. 1** and **2**).[26] They arbitrarily separated patients into those with liver enzymes less than 3 times ULN and more than 3 times ULN. Any elevation in liver enzymes should prompt a thorough history, physical examination, and review of previous laboratory values to help determine the possible etiology of liver injury.

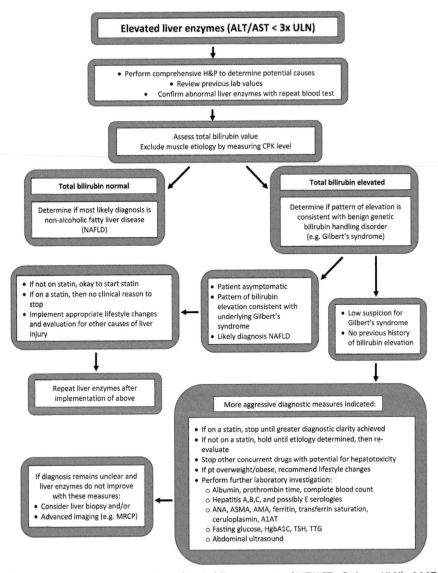

Fig. 1. Comprehensive approach to elevated liver enzymes (ALT/AST <3 times ULN). A1AT, alpha-1 antitrypsin; AMA, anti–mitochondrial antibody; ANA, antinuclear antibody; ASMA, anti–smooth muscle enzyme; CPK, creatine kinase; H&P, history and physical examination; HgbA1C, hemoglobin A1C; MRCP, magnetic resonance cholangiopancreatography; TSH, thyroid-stimulating hormone; TTG, tissue transglutaminase antibodies. (*Adapted from* Bays H, Cohen DE, Chalasani N, Harrison SA, The National Lipid Association's Statin Safety Task Force. An assessment by the Statin Liver Safety Task Force: 2014 update. J Clin Lipidol. 2014 May-Jun;8(3 Suppl):S47-57. PMID: 24793441; with permission.)

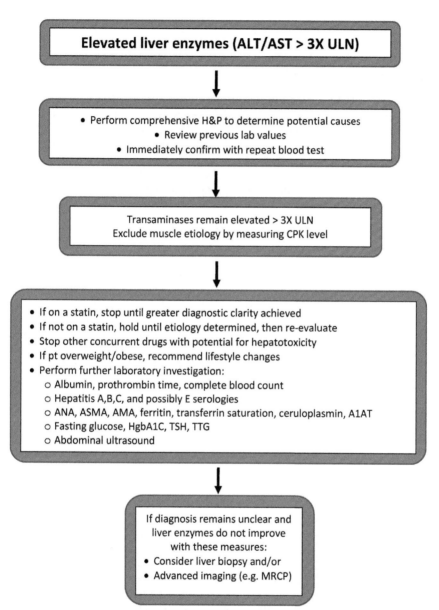

Fig. 2. Comprehensive approach to elevated liver enzymes (ALT/AST >3 times ULN). A1AT, alpha-1 antitrypsin; AMA, anti–mitochondrial antibody; ANA, antinuclear antibody; ASMA, anti–smooth muscle enzyme; CPK, creatine kinase; H&P, history and physical examination; HgbA1C, hemoglobin A1C; MRCP, magnetic resonance cholangiopancreatography; TSH, thyroid stimulating hormone; TTG, tissue transglutaminase antibodies. (*Adapted from* Bays H, Cohen DE, Chalasani N, Harrison SA, The National Lipid Association's Statin Safety Task Force. An assessment by the Statin Liver Safety Task Force: 2014 update. J Clin Lipidol. 2014 May-Jun;8(3 Suppl):S47-57. PMID: 24793441; with permission.)

Liver Enzyme Elevation of Less Than Three Times the Upper Limit of Normal

In patients with confirmed transaminase elevation less than 3 times the ULN and with normal bilirubin and creatine kinase, the next step should involve deciding if the most likely diagnosis is NAFLD. In this clinical scenario, it is okay to start a statin or continue current statin therapy. Liver enzymes should be monitored and other investigation for underlying liver injury investigated. If confirmed transaminase elevation are more than 3 times the ULN but the bilirubin is also elevated, the next step should include evaluation for benign genetic causes of elevation (ie, Gilbert's syndrome). If the patient has a history of periodic asymptomatic elevations in indirect bilirubin consistent with Gilbert's syndrome, then statins can be started or continued. If, in contrast, there is a predominately direct hyperbilirubinemia, statin therapy should be held until the etiology of hyperbilirubinemia is determined based on comprehensive evaluation.[26]

Liver Enzyme Elevation of More Than Three Times the Upper Limit of Normal

If the transaminases are found to be more than 3 times the ULN, the 2014 Statin Liver Safety Task Force recommends immediately repeating the liver enzymes and checking a creatine kinase.[26] If this degree of liver enzyme elevation persists, the statin should be stopped along with any other potential hepatotoxic drugs while a comprehensive evaluation to determine the cause of liver injury is pursued.

Common clinical questions following an episode of statin-related DILI include whether rechallenging is safe, whether a different statin may be used, or if starting the agent at a lower dose should be considered. Data addressing these questions remain extremely limited, and no firm conclusions can be made. The DILIN group could not address these questions from information gathered from their population.[6] One patient was restarted on the same statin and rapidly developed acute injury. None of the patients within this study were switched to a different statin. In the Swedish study, 3 patients were rechallenged with the same statin with a similar pattern of DILI ensuing within 1 month.[15] In 5 cases, a different statin was started after normalization of liver function testing and there was no subsequent development of DILI.

POTENTIAL PREVENTION OF STATIN-INDUCED LIVER INJURY

Bicyclol is a novel synthetic analogue of schiandrin C, an active compound within a Chinese herbal remedy used for the treatment of viral hepatitis.[27] Clinical studies have demonstrated improvement in liver enzymes along with decreased hepatitis inflammation and fibrosis following the administration of oral bicyclol. The proposed mechanism of action involves the reduction in free radical-induced hepatic damage.[28] Naiqiong and colleagues[29] conducted a randomized control trial in China to evaluate the efficacy of bicyclol in the treatment of statin-induced liver injury marking the first trial of its kind. The study included 168 patients with liver injury caused by statins. Treatment with bicyclol compared with polyene phosphatidylcholine (control) resulted in lower ALT levels after 4 weeks of therapy and high rates of transaminase normalization. No serious adverse events were observed and the side effects that were reported did not differ between the 2 groups. Additional studies are needed, but bicyclol may serve as a viable and safe treatment option for mild to moderate DILI related to statins. Mouse models have also demonstrated that beta-glycosphingolipids have a hepatoprotective effect on acetaminophen- and statin-mediated DILI. Researchers suggest that safer drug formulations in the future may include hepatoprotective adjuvants.[30]

USE OF STATINS IN PATIENTS WITH CHRONIC LIVER DISEASE AND CIRRHOSIS

Statins are often underprescribed to those with chronic liver disease owing to the concern for hepatotoxicity, which may not be justified given the rarity of statin associated DILI as discussed elsewhere in this article. There is robust evidence that statin therapy is safe in patients with chronic liver disease, including hepatitis C, and can also be used safely in patients with compensated cirrhosis.[12,31–36] In fact, the 2014 Liver Expert Panel supports that chronic liver disease and compensated cirrhosis are not contraindications to the use of statin therapy.[26] However, statins should not be used in patients with decompensated cirrhosis or acute liver failure.

SPECIAL CONSIDERATION FOR THE USE OF STATINS IN PATIENTS WITH NONALCOHOLIC FATTY LIVER DISEASE

The use of statin therapy is particularly relevant in the setting of NAFLD and nonalcoholic steatohepatitis, given that these patients often have cardiovascular risk factors and hyperlipidemia.[37] A focused investigation of statin use in this population has been undertaken. Two case-control studies evaluated the use of statins in the setting of baseline elevation in transaminases.[33,38] Both studies found that the risk of hepatotoxicity was not increase in those with baseline liver enzymes elevations compared with those with normal baseline liver enzymes. It is postulated that many of the patients in this study population likely had NAFLD, given that there were no other identifiable cause of underlying chronic liver disease. In a small pilot study, Rallidis and colleagues[39] found that liver histology improved with regression of steatosis after 6 months of treatment with pravastatin in patients with biopsy-proven NAFLD. In addition, no significant change in liver enzymes was observed. Another prospective study followed 68 patients with NAFLD for 10 to 16 years and demonstrated that those treated with statin exhibited a significant reduction in liver steatosis when compared with those not prescribed statin therapy.[40] Although these studies are small and lack control groups, the results are encouraging that statin therapy does not lead to more hepatotoxicity in patients with NAFLD and may actually result in improvement of hepatic steatosis.[7,41,42]

Based on the existing evidence, the 2014 Statin Liver Safety Task Force concluded that statins can be safely used in patients with NAFLD and nonalcoholic steatohepatitis.[26,43] The 2018 AASLD practice guidance document on the treatment of NAFLD also concluded that patients with NAFLD or nonalcoholic steatohepatitis can be safely and effectively treated with statins for their dyslipidemia.[44] However, this document did not recommend specifically treating NAFLD with statins in patients without dyslipidemia.

POTENTIAL HEPATIC BENEFITS OF STATINS

There are some preclinical data and clinical studies suggesting that statins may have direct beneficial effects on the liver.[45,46] Recent studies have demonstrated that endothelial expression of the transcription factor Kruppel-like factor 2 and its subsequent vasoprotective targets improve vascular dysfunction in cirrhotic livers. Statins have been shown to upregulate Kruppel-like factor 2 in rat models, conferring endothelial protection with potential to improve portal hypertension and possibly reduce hepatic fibrosis.[47–51] Other studies have also demonstrated deceases in portal hypertension with statin treatment in animal models.[52,53] Rat models of ischemia–reperfusion injury have also revealed that statin therapy may protect against both renal and hepatic injury.[54–56]

Statins are safe in patients with chronic viral hepatitis and may also confer additional benefit. A small study of 31 veterans showed that fluvastatin as monotherapy resulted in suppression of hepatitis C viremia and no worsening liver tests.[57] A large cohort study of patients with chronic hepatitis B in Taiwan found that those who received statin therapy had a dose-dependent reduction in the risk of cirrhosis and subsequent decompensation.[58]

SUMMARY

Idiosyncratic DILI is a well-described but uncommon side effect of statin use. Up to 3% of patients on statins may develop elevated liver enzymes. However, the risk of clinically significant liver injury is rare. This risk should not overshadow the cardiovascular benefits when treatment is indicated. Measurement of liver enzymes should be performed before initiating statin therapy; however, routine monitoring is not necessary in the absence of clinical signs or symptoms, suggesting possible hepatotoxicity. In this article, we have presented diagnostic and therapeutic algorithms for patients with possible statin-induced DILI. There is not enough data to guide management decisions such as rechallenging patients with statin-induced DILI with the same statin, switching to a different statin, or using a lower dose. Statins may be used safely in those patients with stable chronic liver disease, including those individuals with NAFLD, chronic hepatitis C, and compensated cirrhosis. Statin use should be avoided in those with suspected DILI related to statin therapy when transaminases are greater than 3 times the ULN or when hyperbilirubinemia unrelated to Gilbert's syndrome is present. Statin therapy should also be avoided in significant acute liver injury, liver failure, and decompensated cirrhosis. In addition to their beneficial effects for patients with CAD and dyslipidemia, statins may actually offer some direct hepatoprotective benefits including, a decrease in fibrosis and portal hypertension; however, further clinical studies are needed.

REFERENCES

1. Sirtori CR. The pharmacology of statins. Pharmacol Res 2014;88:3–11.
2. Taylor F, Huffman MD, Macedo AF, et al. Statins for the primary prevention of cardiovascular disease. Cochrane Database Syst Rev 2013;(1):CD004816.
3. Guyton JR, Bays HE, Grundy SM, et al, The National Lipid Association Statin Intolerance Panel. An assessment by the Statin Intolerance Panel: 2014 update. J Clin Lipidol 2014;8(3 Suppl):S72–81.
4. Bełtowski J, Wójcicka G, Jamroz-Wiśniewska A. Adverse effects of statins - mechanisms and consequences. Curr Drug Saf 2009;4(3):209–28.
5. Ramkumar S, Raghunath A, Raghunath S. Statin therapy: review of safety and potential side effects. Acta Cardiol Sin 2016;32(6):631–9.
6. Russo MW, Hoofnagle JH, Gu J, et al. Spectrum of statin hepatotoxicity: experience of the drug-induced liver injury network. Hepatology 2014;60(2):679–86.
7. Chalasani N. Statins and hepatotoxicity: focus on patients with fatty liver. Hepatology 2005;41(4):690–5.
8. de Denus S, Spinler SA, Miller K, et al. Statins and liver toxicity: a meta-analysis. Pharmacotherapy 2004;24(5):584–91.
9. Newman C, Tsai J, Szarek M, et al. Comparative safety of atorvastatin 80 mg versus 10 mg derived from analysis of 49 completed trials in 14,236 patients. Am J Cardiol 2006;97(1):61–7.

10. Alsheikh-Ali AA, Maddukuri PV, Han H, et al. Effect of the magnitude of lipid lowering on risk of elevated liver enzymes, rhabdomyolysis, and cancer: insights from large randomized statin trials. J Am Coll Cardiol 2007;50(5):409–18.

11. Kasliwal R, Wilton LV, Cornelius V, et al. Safety profile of rosuvastatin: results of a prescription-event monitoring study of 11,680 patients. Drug Saf 2007;30(2): 157–70.

12. Sniderman AD. Is there value in liver function test and creatine phosphokinase monitoring with statin use? Am J Cardiol 2004;94(9A):30F–4F.

13. Björnsson ES, Bergmann OM, Helgi K, et al. Incidence, presentation, and outcomes in patients with drug-induced liver injury in the general population of Iceland. Gastroenterology 2013;144(7):1419–25.

14. Björnsson E, Olsson R. Outcome and prognostic markers in severe drug-induced liver disease. Hepatology 2005;42(2):481–9.

15. Björnsson E, Jacobsen EI, Kalaitzakis E. Hepatotoxicity associated with statins: reports of idiosyncratic liver injury post-marketing. J Hepatol 2012;56(2):374–80.

16. Perdices EV, Medina-Cáliz I, Hernando S, et al. Hepatotoxicity associated with statin use: analysis of the cases included in the Spanish Hepatotoxicity Registry. Rev Esp Enferm Dig 2014;106(4):246–54.

17. Medina-Caliz I, Robles-Diaz M, Garcia-Muñoz B, et al. Definition and risk factors for chronicity following acute idiosyncratic drug-induced liver injury. J Hepatol 2016;65:532–42.

18. Temple R. Hy's law: predicting serious hepatotoxicity. Pharmacoepidemiol Drug Saf 2006;15:241–3.

19. Russo MW, Galanko JA, Shrestha R, et al. Liver transplantation for acute liver failure from drug induced liver injury in the United States. Liver Transpl 2004;10(8): 1018–23.

20. Haque T, Sasatomi E, Hayashi PH. Drug-induced liver injury: pattern recognition and future directions. Gut Liver 2016;10(1):27–36.

21. Nakayama S, Murashima N. Overlap syndrome of autoimmune hepatitis and primary biliary cirrhosis triggered by fluvastatin. Indian J Gastroenterol 2011; 30(2):97–9.

22. Pelli N, Setti M, Ceppa P, et al. Autoimmune hepatitis revealed by atorvastatin. Eur J Gastroenterol Hepatol 2003;15(8):921–4.

23. U.S. Food and Drug Administration. Drug database. Available at: https://www. accessdata.fda.gov/scripts/cder/daf/index.cfm. Accessed February 10, 2019.

24. Cohen DE, Anania FA, Chalasani N, National Lipid Association Statin Safety Task Force Liver Expert Panel. An assessment of statin safety by hepatologists. Am J Cardiol 2006;97(8A):77C–81C.

25. US Food and Drug Administration. FDA drug safety communication: important safety label changes to cholesterol-lowering statin drugs. Available at: http:// www.fda.gov/drugs/drugsafety/ucm293101.htm. Accessed February 2, 2019.

26. Bays H, Cohen DE, Chalasani N, et al, The National Lipid Association's Statin Safety Task Force. An assessment by the Statin Liver Safety Task Force: 2014 update. J Clin Lipidol 2014;8(3 Suppl):S47–57.

27. Liu GT. Bicyclol: a novel drug for treating chronic viral hepatitis B and C. Med Chem 2009;5(1):29–43.

28. Liu GT, Li Y, Wei HL, et al. Mechanism of protective action of bicyclol against CCl4-induced liver injury in mice. Liver Int 2005;25(4):872–9.

29. Naiqiong W, Liansheng W, Zhanying H, et al. A multicenter and randomized controlled trial of bicyclol in the treatment of statin-induced liver injury. Med Sci Monit 2017;23:5760–6.

30. Mizrahi M, Adar T, Lalazar G, et al. Glycosphingolipids prevent APAP and HMG-CoA reductase inhibitors-mediated liver damage: a novel method for "safer drug" formulation that prevents drug-induced liver injury. J Clin Transl Hepatol 2018;6(2):127–34.

31. Moctezuma-Velázquez C, Abraldes JG, Montano-Loza AJ. The use of statins in patients with chronic liver disease and cirrhosis. Curr Treat Options Gastroenterol 2018;16(2):226–40.

32. Segarra-Newnham M, Parra D, Martin-Cooper EM. Effectiveness and hepatotoxicity of statins in men seropositive for hepatitis C virus. Pharmacotherapy 2007; 27(6):845–51.

33. Vuppalanchi R, Chalasani N. Statins for hyperlipidemia in patients with chronic liver disease: are they safe? Clin Gastroenterol Hepatol 2006;4(7):838–9.

34. Khorashadi S, Hasson NK, Cheung RC. Incidence of statin hepatotoxicity in patients with hepatitis C. Clin Gastroenterol Hepatol 2006;4(7):902–7.

35. Avins AL, Manos MM, Ackerson L, et al. Hepatic effects of lovastatin exposure in patients with liver disease: a retrospective cohort study. Drug Saf 2008;31(4): 325–34.

36. Chang CH, Chang YC, Lee YC, et al. Severe hepatic injury associated with different statins in patients with chronic liver disease: a nationwide population-based cohort study. J Gastroenterol Hepatol 2015;30(1):155–62.

37. Francque SM, van der Graaff D, Kwanten WJ. Non-alcoholic fatty liver disease and cardiovascular risk: pathophysiological mechanisms and implications. J Hepatol 2016;65(2):425–43.

38. Chalasani N, Aljadhey H, Kesterson J, et al. Patients with elevated liver enzymes are not at higher risk for statin hepatotoxicity. Gastroenterology 2004;128: 1287–92.

39. Rallidis LS, Drakoulis CK, Parasi AS. Pravastatin in patients with nonalcoholic steatohepatitis: results of a pilot study. Atherosclerosis 2004;174(1):193–6.

40. Ekstedt M, Franzén LE, Mathiesen UL, et al. Statins in non-alcoholic fatty liver disease and chronically elevated liver enzymes: a histopathological follow-up study. J Hepatol 2007;47(1):135–41.

41. Eslami L, Merat S, Malekzadeh R, et al. Statins for non-alcoholic fatty liver disease and non-alcoholic steatohepatitis. Cochrane Database Syst Rev 2013;(12):CD008623.

42. Athyros VG, Boutari C, Stavropoulos K, et al. Statins: an under-appreciated asset for the prevention and the treatment of NAFLD or NASH and the related cardio-vascular risk. Curr Vasc Pharmacol 2018;16(3):246–53.

43. Riley P, Al Bakir M, O'Donohue J, et al. Prescribing statins to patients with nonalcoholic fatty liver disease: real cardiovascular benefits outweigh theoretical hepatotoxic risk. Cardiovasc Ther 2009;27(3):216–20.

44. Chalasani N, Younossi Z, Lavine JE, et al. The diagnosis and management of nonalcoholic fatty liver disease: practice guidance from the American Association for the study of liver diseases. Hepatology 2018;67(1):328–57.

45. Vargas JI, Arrese M, Shah VH, et al. Use of statins in patients with chronic liver disease and cirrhosis: current views and prospects. Curr Gastroenterol Rep 2017;19(9):43.

46. Imprialos KP, Stavropoulos K, Doumas M, et al. The potential role of statins in treating liver disease. Expert Rev Gastroenterol Hepatol 2018;12(4):331–9.

47. Gracia-Sancho J, Russo L, García-Calderó H, et al. Endothelial expression of transcription factor Kruppel-like factor 2 and its vasoprotective target genes in the normal and cirrhotic rat liver. Gut 2011;60(4):517–24.

48. Marrone G, Russo L, Rosado E, et al. The transcription factor KLF2 mediates hepatic endothelial protection and paracrine endothelial-stellate cell deactivation induced by statins. J Hepatol 2013;58(1):98–103.
49. Marrone G, Maeso-Díaz R, García-Cardena G, et al. KLF2 exerts antifibrotic and vasoprotective effects in cirrhotic rat livers: behind the molecular mechanisms of statins. Gut 2015;64(9):1434–43.
50. Zafra C, Abraldes JG, Turnes J, et al. Simvastatin enhances hepatic nitric oxide production and decreases the hepatic vascular tone in patients with cirrhosis. Gastroenterology 2004;126(3):749–55.
51. El-Ashmawy NE, El-Bahrawy HA, Shamloula MM, et al. Antifibrotic effect of AT-1 blocker and statin in rats with hepatic fibrosis. Clin Exp Pharmacol Physiol 2015; 42(9):979–87.
52. Arab JP, Shah VH. Statins and portal hypertension: a tale of two models. Hepatology 2016;63:2044–7.
53. Abraldes JG, Albillos A, Bañares R, et al. Simvastatin lowers portal pressure in patients with cirrhosis and portal hypertension: a randomized controlled trial. Gastroenterology 2009;136(5):1651–8.
54. Alexandropoulos D, Bazigos GV, Doulamis IP, et al. Protective effects of N-acetyl-cysteine and atorvastatin against renal and hepatic injury in a rat model of intestinal ischemia-reperfusion. Biomed Pharmacother 2017;89:673–80.
55. Cámara-Lemarroy CR, Guzmán-de la Garza FJ, Alarcón-Galván G, et al. Hepatic ischemia/reperfusion injury is diminished by atorvastatin in Wistar rats. Arch Med Res 2014;45(3):210–6.
56. Kocak FE, Kucuk A, Ozyigit F, et al. Protective effects of simvastatin administered in the experimental hepatic ischemia-reperfusion injury rat model. J Surg Res 2015;199(2):393–401.
57. Bader T, Fazili J, Madhoun M, et al. Fluvastatin inhibits hepatitis C replication in humans. Am J Gastroenterol 2008;103(6):1383–9.
58. Huang Y-W, Lee C-L, Yang S-S, et al. Statins reduce the risk of cirrhosis and its decompensation in chronic hepatitis B patients: a nationwide cohort study. Am J Gastroenterol 2016;111:976–85.

Drug-Induced Liver Injury in the Setting of Analgesic Use

Umar Darr, MD[a], Norman Leslie Sussman, MD[b],*

KEYWORDS

- Analgesic • Acetaminophen • NSAIDs • Opiates • Acute liver injury
- Acute liver failure • Liver transplantation

KEY POINTS

- Acetaminophen (APAP) at high doses is toxic and remains the most common cause of acute liver failure in western countries. Timely N-acetylcysteine prevents or reduces liver injury.
- Non-APAP nonsteroidal antiinflammatory drugs, despite their widespread use, rarely cause liver injury.
- Opiate-APAP combination drugs were previously a major source of APAP overdose. This problem has been alleviated by Food and Drug Administration–mandated reduced APAP dosing in these combination products.
- Tricyclic antidepressants may be used as adjunctive therapy and are rarely associated with liver injury.
- Anticonvulsants such as gabapentin and pregabalin are commonly used for diabetic neuropathy and rarely cause liver injury.

INTRODUCTION

Pain is one of the most common reasons for unscheduled physician visits,[1] and antiinflammatory and analgesic medications are among the most popular drugs in household medicine chests across America. In 2016, an estimated 11% to 40% of the United States population complained of chronic pain.[2] Health care professionals find themselves balancing patient demands for pain relief with the adverse effects of prescribed and self-administered analgesics. Revenue in analgesics amounted to approximately $5.2 billion in 2018 and is expected to grow by 2.2% annually.[3]

Analgesics include a diverse group of compounds from multiple drug classes (**Table 1**). Acetaminophen (APAP) is toxic in high doses and is the most common

[a] Houston Methodist Medical Center, 16605 Southwest Freeway, Suite 175, MOB 3, Sugar Land, TX 77479, USA; [b] Baylor College of Medicine, 6620 Main Street, Suite 1425, Houston, TX 77030, USA
* Corresponding author.
E-mail address: normans@bcm.edu

Clin Liver Dis 24 (2020) 121–129
https://doi.org/10.1016/j.cld.2019.09.008
1089-3261/20/© 2019 Elsevier Inc. All rights reserved.

Table 1
Nonsteroidal antiinflammatory drugs and hepatotoxicity

Drug	Mechanism	Onset	Manifestation	Market Status (USA)
Aspirin	Dose dependent	Days to weeks	Hepatocellular, Reye syndrome	Available
Indomethacin	Metabolic	1–7 mo	Hepatocellular dysfunction, variable cholestasis	Available
Sulindac	Hypersensitivity	≤8 wk	Mixed hepatocellular damage/cholestasis, hypersensitivity reaction	Available
Ibuprofen	Metabolic	1–12 wk	Mixed hepatocellular damage/cholestasis, Stevens-Johnson syndrome	Available
Naproxen	Metabolic	≤12 wk	Cholestasis	Available
Diclofenac	Metabolic/immunologic	1–3 mo	Mixed hepatocellular damage/cholestasis, hypersensitivity syndrome	Available
Nimesulide	Metabolic	≤6 mo	Cholestasis	Not available
COXIBs	Metabolic		Mixed hepatocellular damage/cholestasis	Some available
Oxicams	Metabolic	1–5 wk	Mixed hepatocellular damage/cholestasis, massive and submassive necrosis, and ductopenia	Available

single cause of acute liver failure in western nations[4]; severe cases may be fatal or may require liver transplantation. APAP-opiate or opioid combinations are declining in popularity but were responsible for at least 50% of serious APAP-related liver injury cases in the United States.[4,5] Non-APAP compounds are generally safe but may cause liver injury or cholestasis. The numerous variations of opioid and nonopioid as well as inflammatory and noninflammatory analgesics make attempts to curb liver toxicity difficult to achieve. This article focuses on common analgesic agents including acetaminophen, nonsteroidal antiinflammatory drugs (NSAIDs), opioids, tricyclic antidepressants (TCAs), anticonvulsants, and combination drugs.

ACETAMINOPHEN

APAP is one of the most widely used analgesics in the United States.[6] It is safe at a therapeutic dose, usually defined in adults as up to 4 g per day. Surprisingly, an elevated alanine aminotransferase (ALT) level greater than 3 times the upper limit of normal was seen in 33% to 44% of normal volunteers who were administered 4 g of APAP daily for 14 days.[7] ALT returned to normal on stopping APAP, and no liver impairment was reported. In contrast, high-dose APAP is reliably hepatotoxic and is the most common cause of acute liver failure (ALF) in the United States, comprising approximately half of all cases.[4–6] The chance of recovery from APAP-induced ALF is higher than that from other causes, but severe injury may be fatal unless that patient is rescued by liver transplantation.

APAP/narcotic combinations became popular because of the perception that patients would take lower doses of narcotics. Instead, patients seeking pain relief frequently ignored the APAP dose. In 2010, more than 131 million combination

APAP-hydrocodone prescriptions were written and at least 6% percent of them exceeded the 4 g maximum daily dose.[8] In addition, APAP-opioid combination products have contributed to 63% of total overdoses in the United States.[9] In attempting to curb this trend, the Food and Drug Administration (FDA) of the United States has limited the APAP dose to a maximum of 325 mg per tablet in combination products.[10]

APAP toxicity is a multistep process (**Fig. 1**). The bulk of ingested APAP is rendered nontoxic by conjugation, but about 5% is converted to a toxic benzoquinoneimine metabolite (N-acetyl-p-benzoquinone imine [NAPQI]) by CYP2E1.[11] In subtoxic doses, NAPQI is rendered harmless by conjugation to glutathione, which is usually abundant in hepatocytes. Toxicity occurs when intracellular glutathione stores are depleted, a situation seen in fasting, malnutrition, and chronic excessive alcohol ingestion. In a low glutathione state, NAPQI binds to cysteine residues in cellular proteins and causes cell necrosis. Disrupted cells release their content into the circulation, resulting in characteristically elevated AST and ALT levels in blood, usually 24 to 48 hours after ingestion (**Fig. 2**). Also released at the time of cell necrosis are APAP adducts that are unique to APAP-induced liver injury.[12] APAP adducts can be measured by high-performance liquid chromatography,[13] and a recently described immunoassay promises to make this a point of care test to identify APAP-induced injury when evaluating patients with acute liver failure.[14,15]

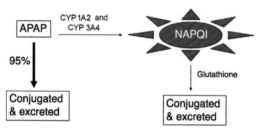

Fig. 1. Acetaminophen (APAP) toxicity is a multistep process. First, most APAP is rendered harmless by conjugated. Second, a small but variable fraction is converted to the toxic metabolite N-acetyl-p-benzoquinone imine (NAPQI). Third, NAPQI is rendered nontoxic by binding to glutathione (GSH). Fourth, NAPQI damages hepatocytes when GSH is depleted.

Diagnosis of Acetaminophen Toxicity

Most of the 60,000 annual cases of APAP overdose in the United States result in minor liver injury; only 500 to 1000 go on to acute liver failure.[16] The Acute Liver Failure Study Group reported that cases were divided about equally between intentional and accidental overdose with about 60% from APAP-narcotic preparations.[9]

APAP toxicity should be suspected in anyone who states he/she has ingested an excessive APAP dose or who presents with a characteristic clinical picture (**Table 2**). APAP is rapidly cleared from the circulation with a half-life of 2 to 3 hours after reaching its peak concentration.[17] Because of this short half-life, APAP levels are rarely detectable at the time of liver injury. A detectable APAP level at the time of liver injury indicates either ongoing ingestion or overdose with a sustained release formulation. This is an important finding that indicates a need for a longer course of the antidote, N-acetylcysteine (NAC).

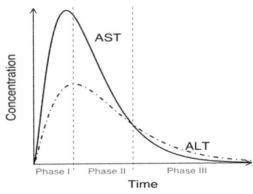

Fig. 2. Hypothetical decay curves for AST and ALT after acute liver injury. After acute injury, blood levels of AST and ALT increase rapidly. At their peak, AST concentration is twice the concentration of ALT. Provided no further injury occurs, AST will clear at about 50% every 24 hours, and AST will clear at about 33% every 24 hours. The dynamic AST:ALT ratio was used as a factor to calculate the risk of death after APAP overdose using a series of differential equations. (*Courtesy of* Chris Remien, PhD.)

Treatment of Acetaminophen Toxicity

Activated charcoal (AC) may be effectively used in addition to NAC within the first few hours of ingestion.[18] Because most liver units see patients well beyond 24 hours after ingestion, AC is rarely used.

Table 2
Clinical features of acetaminophen overdose

Feature	Comment
Elevated AST and ALT levels	AST and ALT may be very high—frequently >5000 IU/L AST concentration is twice ALT at peak AST and ALT clear at predictable rates
Elevated INR	Usually very high—out of proportion to the severity of liver injury Not usually associated with increased risk of bleeding
Total bilirubin <5 mg/dL	Bilirubin $\geq$5 suggests an alternative cause
Hepatic encephalopathy (HE)	HE distinguishes acute liver failure (ALF) from acute liver injury (ALI) Prognosis is worse for patients with HE
Elevated creatinine	Variable finding—worse prognosis in patients with renal injury May be secondary to liver injury or direct toxicity of APAP
Acidosis	A typical finding at presentation Persistent acidosis after volume replacement is associated with a worse outcome
APAP level	Usually undetectable at the onset of liver injury Detectable APAP indicates massive overdose, ongoing ingestion, or overdose with a sustained-release formulation
APAP adducts	Compound that is found exclusively in APAP toxicity Not currently available, but a rapid test is in development

Abbreviation: INR, international normalized ratio.

Irrespective of timing, NAC should be given immediately if APAP poisoning is suspected. Early administration may prevent liver injury, and later administration may limit liver necrosis. The suggested protocol for a proprietary IV NAC product (Acetadote, Cumberland Pharmaceuticals Inc. Nashville, TN 37203) is a 3-bag method that includes the following:

- Loading dose (150 mg/kg in 200 mL 5% dextrose over 1 hour)
- Second dose (50 mg/kg in 500 mL 5% dextrose over 4 hours)
- Third dose (100 mg/kg in 1000 mL 5% dextrose over 16 hours)

The value of further dosing is uncertain, but some centers recommend extending the third dose for an additional 16 to 32 hours.

Additional steps in managing APAP overdose are shown in **Table 3** and have been discussed elsewhere in more detail.[19]

Table 3 Management of acetaminophen overdose	
Intervention	**Rationale**
Activated charcoal	Useful if the patient reports recent APAP ingestion
N-acetylcysteine (NAC)	Administer immediately for all suspected cases of APAP overdose
Start IV glucose (5%–10%)	Check blood sugar every hour—hypoglycemia is a lethal complication of acute liver failure. Do not use 50% glucose push
Replace phosphorus	Hypophosphatemia is a lethal complication during liver regeneration. Check at least twice daily
Head of bed elevation	Elevated to 20° and avoid stimulation
Monitor liver tests	Every 24 h is sufficient

NONSTEROIDAL ANTIINFLAMMATORY DRUGS

An estimated 17 million Americans take NSAIDs every day. The incidence of NSAID-induced liver injury ranges from 1 to 9 cases in 100,000 persons and comprises roughly 10% of total reported drug-induced hepatotoxicity.[20] Liver injury typically presents within 1 to 3 months. Liver injury is idiosyncratic rather than intrinsic. It is thought that toxicity is linked to increased hepatobiliary drug concentrations resulting in reactive metabolites, oxidative stress, and mitochondrial injury. Most NSAIDs share similar therapeutic antiinflammatory and antipyretic properties, including adverse effects. Its symptoms range from asymptomatic liver disease to acute liver failure.[21]

Aspirin

The advent of aspirin marked the beginning of the NSAIDs era. It functions as a noncompetitive irreversible inhibitor of both cyclooxygenase 1 and 2 (COX-1, COX-2) and is further metabolized to salicylate and other compounds by hepatocytes. Aspirin hepatotoxicity is often mild and reversible. Liver injury is most commonly described in patients with chronic aspirin therapy, defined as at least 6 days of use before toxic onset.[22]

Clinical and pathologic spectrums range from acute self-limited disease to cholestatic hepatitis and acute liver failure. Symptoms may include allergic features such as rash and fever, and the diagnosis is usually made with elevated liver tests in the setting of a high serum salicylate level. Toxicity is more likely in those consuming more than 100 mg/kg per day and/or with salicylate levels greater than 25 mg/dL. Most of the toxic cases will have a normal total bilirubin and an AST less than 500 IU/L. Biopsy findings may show periportal and lobular necroinflammation, autoimmune hepatitis, or granulomatous hepatitis.[22]

Treatment is withdrawal of therapy. Resolution of hepatotoxicity, even with severe injury, is typical. Reexposure to aspirin after resolution of hepatotoxicity is safe at lower dosing.[22]

Aspirin was commonly associated with Reye syndrome, with 90% of cases occurring in children. The incidence of Reye syndrome declined in the 1980s after a campaign alerted the public to the dangers of using aspirin as an antipyretic in young children. Reye syndrome is not related to blood salicylate levels, but seems to have a genetic basis, and may (rarely) occur in a patient who has not taken aspirin. The incidences of Reye syndrome since public health efforts have declined with no more than 2 cases reported annually since 1994.[23]

Diclofenac

Diclofenac-induced liver injury is almost exclusively hepatocellular. Enzyme abnormalities have been reported in approximately 15% of chronic users but rarely greater than 3 times the upper limit of normal.[24] The severity of diclofenac toxicity is debated. A recent meta-analysis reported that diclofenac has the highest rates of hepatotoxicity among all NSAIDs (ref). On the contrary, the Multinational Etoricoxib and Diclofenac Arthritis Long-Term Study Program (MEDAL Program), the longest and largest diclofenac liver–related study database, reported an incidence of diclofenac liver–related hospitalizations as 16 per 100,000 patient years. In addition, only 0.023% of cases fulfilled Hy's law, indicating low liver toxicity rates associated with diclofenac.[25]

Sulindac

Sulindac is associated with a 5 to 10 times increased incidence of hepatotoxicity compared with other NSAIDs. Its antiapoptotic effect once made it very popular in colonic polyposis treatment. Hepatotoxicity is via hypersensitivity. Symptoms are typically fever, rash, nausea, and vomiting arising within a few days of initiation. Enzyme elevation is usually hepatocellular or mixed. Recovery is rapid with drug cessation. Sulindac-induced acute liver injury is well known, but rare and self-limited.[21,26,27]

Ibuprofen

Ibuprofen's antiinflammatory, analgesic, and antipyretic properties have made it one of the most commonly used NSADs worldwide. It was first introduced in the UK market in 1969. Low rates of gastrointestinal adverse events compared with other NSAIDs have made it a popular choice in patients suffering from arthritis. Short half-life and lack of pathologic downstream metabolites may explain its safety profile. Limited reported cases have suggested a possible increased liver injury risk in patients with hepatitis C. Consensus remains that ibuprofen has the safest liver profile among all NSAIDs.[21,28]

COX-2 Inhibitors

COX-2 inhibitors (COXIBs) selectively inhibit cycloxygenase-2 (COX-2), an enzyme responsible for inflammation and pain. They have, as ibuprofen, gained popularity due to their gastrointestinal safety profile compared with nonselective NSAIDs. Laine and colleagues[29] published a comprehensive evaluation of COX-2 inhibitors in patients with osteoarthritis. Despite its useful effects, significant controversy includes its cardiovascular adverse events such as increased myocardial infarction and arterial hypertension. Valdecoxib, rofecoxib, and lumiracoxib were removed from the market in 2004 and 2005, respectively.[21]

Oxicams

Oxicams are nonselective COX inhibitors with the exception of meloxicam, which has a preference for COX-2. General consensus holds that hepatotoxicity is uncommon. Piroxicam has the strongest association with hepatocellular necrosis, hepatocanalicular cholestasis, and ductopenia. Hepatotoxicity was reported with isoxicam and droxicam, but reports are sporadic and not validated.[20]

Nimesulide

Similar to COXIBs, nimesulide has analgesic, antiinflammatory, and antipyretic activities secondary to its effect on COX-2. It also includes a relatively safe gastrointestinal profile. Since 1997, reports have confirmed severe forms of liver toxicity resulting in death and/or liver transplantation in as little as 3 days postingestion. Despite overall low incidence, nimesulide is not FDA approved and is unavailable in the United States. It remains on the market in European.[21]

OPIOIDS

Opioid side effects include sedation, constipation, and precipitation of encephalopathy. Drug clearance is reduced in patients with liver disease, potentially leading to accentuated opiate effects.[30] Mild pain that is not well controlled with acetaminophen may be best managed with either low-dose tramadol or immediate release oxycodone—more potent opiates and opioids such as morphine and hydromorphone should be used as last-line alternatives. Assessment for constipation is important, and laxatives should be initiated if necessary.

Despite the necessary caution, opioids rarely cause drug-induced liver disease. Rather, cardiorespiratory failure from overdose is the primary cause of death.[31]

As stated previously, fixed drug combinations with acetaminophen may cause APAP-related toxicity, especially in presence of opioid abuse. This has led to the FDA recommendations against the use of high-dose APAP-opioid combinations.[10]

ADJUVANT ANALGESICS

TCAs such as amitriptyline are the recommended first-line treatments for neuropathic pain in patients suffering from poorly controlled diabetes. In cirrhosis, reduction of TCA clearance by CYP450 increases the risk for toxicity. Anticholinergic effects and drowsiness are common and may be accentuated in patients with hepatic insufficiency. Nortriptyline is an effective alternative for neuropathic pain with fewer adverse effects. TCA therapy should be started at the lowest dose with gradual titration.[31]

Anticonvulsant agents and serotonin-norepinephrine reuptake inhibitors (SNRI) have been used to treat trigeminal neuralgia and neuropathy. Desvenlafaxine may be better tolerated in patients with liver disease as it is not metabolized by the enzyme CYP450, providing an alternative to commonly used SNRI's such as duloxetine and venlafaxine. Second generation anti-epileptics including gabapentin and pregabalin also do not undergo extensive hepatic metabolism making them relatively safe methods for pain relief.[31]

SUMMARY

Providing safe and effective analgesia to patients with or without chronic liver disease can be challenging. No consensus guidelines aid clinicians in initiating or monitoring analgesic use, and over-the-counter drugs are frequently used without the clinician's knowledge or advice. Clinicians should be aware of the toxic potential of APAP in all patients and the possibility of slowed clearance of certain drugs in patients with impaired liver function.

REFERENCES

1. St Sauver JL, Warner DO, Yawn BP, et al. Why patients visit their doctors: assessing the most prevalent conditions in a defined American population. Mayo Clin Proc 2013;88(1):56–67.
2. Dahlhamer J, Lucas J, Zelaya C, et al. Prevalence of chronic pain and high-impact chronic pain among adults — United States, 2016. MMWR Morb Mortal Wkly Rep 2018;67:1001–6.
3. Statista. Analgesic revenue and average revenue per capita. Available at: https://www.statista.com/outlook/18010000/109/analgesics/united-states#market-revenue. Accessed April 8, 2019.
4. Yoon E, Babar A, Choudhary M, et al. Acetaminophen-induced hepatotoxicity: a comprehensive update. J Clin Transl Hepatol 2016;4:131.
5. Michna E, Duh MS, Korves C, et al. Removal of opioid/acetaminophen combination prescription pain medications: assessing the evidence for hepatotoxicity and consequences of removal of these medications. Pain Med 2010;11:369.
6. Lee WM. Acetaminophen and the U.S. Acute liver failure study group: lowering the risks of hepatic failure. Hepatology 2004;40:6.
7. Watkins PB, Kaplowitz N, Slattery JT, et al. Aminotransferase elevations in healthy adults receiving 4 grams of acetaminophen daily: a randomized controlled trial. JAMA 2006;296:87–93.
8. Clark R, Fisher JE, Sketris IS, et al. Population prevalence of high dose paracetamol in dispensed paracetamol/opioid prescription combinations: an observational study. BMC Clin Pharmacol 2012;12:11.
9. Larson AM, Polson J, Fontana RJ, et al. Acetaminophen-induced acute liver failure: results of a United States multicenter, prospective study. Hepatology 2005; 42:1364.
10. United States Food and Drug Administration. FDA Drug Safety Communication: Prescription Acetaminophen Products to be Limited to 325 mg Per Dosage Unit; Boxed Warning Will Highlight Potential for Severe Liver Failure. 2018. Available at: https://www.fda.gov/drugs/drug-safety-and-availability/fda-drug-safety-communication-prescription-acetaminophen-products-be-limited-325-mg-dosage-unit. Accessed April 8, 2019.
11. Mazaleuskaya LL, Sangkuhl K, Thorn CF, et al. PharmGKB summary: pathways of acetaminophen metabolism at the therapeutic versus toxic doses. Pharmacogenet Genomics 2015;25(8):416–26.
12. James LP, Letzig L, Simpson PM, et al. Pharmacokinetics of acetaminophen-protein adducts in adults with acetaminophen overdose and acute liver failure. Drug Metab Dispos 2009;37:1779–84.
13. Davern TJ 2nd, James LP, Hinson JA, et al. Measurement of serum acetaminophen-protein adducts in patients with acute liver failure. Gastroenterology 2006;130:687–94.

14. Roberts DW, Lee WM, Hinson JA, et al. An immunoassay to rapidly measure acetaminophen protein adducts accurately identifies patients with acute liver injury or failure. Clin Gastroenterol Hepatol 2017;15(4):555–62.e3.
15. Sussman NL, Remien CH. The headache of acetaminophen overdose: getting the NAC. Clin Gastroenterol Hepatol 2017;15:563–4.
16. Fontana RJ. Acute liver failure including acetaminophen overdose. Med Clin North Am 2008;92(4):761–94, viii.
17. US Pharm. Acetaminophen toxicity: what pharmacists need to know. 2014;39(3):HS2–8.
18. Spiller HA, Winter ML, Klein-Schwartz W, et al. Efficacy of activated charcoal administered more than four hours after acetaminophen overdose. J Emerg Med 2006;30:1.
19. Wallace CI, Dargan PI, Jones AL. Paracetamol overdose: an evidence based flowchart to guide management. Emerg Med J 2002;19:202.
20. Bessone F. Non-steroidal anti-inflammatory drugs: what is the actual risk of liver damage? World J Gastroenterol 2010;16(45):5651–61.
21. Boelsterli UA. Mechanisms of NSAID-induced hepatotoxicity: focus on nimesulide. Drug Saf 2002;25:633–48.
22. Garber E, Craig RM, Bahu RM. Letter: aspirin hepatotoxicity. Ann Intern Med 1975;82:592.
23. Chapman J, Arnold JK. Reye syndrome. In: StatPearls. Treasure Island (FL): StatPearls Publishing; 2019. Available at: https://www.ncbi.nlm.nih.gov/books/NBK526101/.
24. LiverTox database. Diclofenac. Available at: https://livertox.nih.gov/Diclofenac.htm#reference. Accessed April 9, 2019.
25. Cannon P, Christopher. (2006). Multinational etoricoxib and diclofenac arthritis long-term (MEDAL) study program: Cardiovascular outcomes following long-term treatment with etoricoxib versus diclofenac in patients with osteoarthritis and rheumatoid arthritis. The Lancet; 2424-2424.
26. LiverTox database. Sulindac. Available at: https://livertox.nlm.nih.gov/Sulindac.htm. Accessed April 9, 2019.
27. Matsuhashi N, Nakajima A, Fukushima Y, et al. Effects of sulindac on sporadic colorectal adenomatous polyps. Gut 1997;40(3):344–9.
28. Rainsford KD. Ibuprofen: pharmacology, efficacy and safety. Inflammopharmacology 2009;17:275–342.
29. Laine L, White WB, Rostom A, Hochberg M. COX-2 Selective Inhibitors in the Treatment of Osteoarthritis. Semin Arthritis Rheum 2008;38(3):165–87.
30. Tegeder I, Lötsch J, Geisslinger G. Pharmacokinetics of opioids in liver disease. Clin Pharmacokinet 1999;37:17.
31. Dwyer JP, Jayasekera C, Nicoll A. Analgesia in cirrhosis. J Gastroenterol Hepatol 2014;29:1356–60.

Drug-Induced Liver Injury Resources and Reporting for the Clinician

Marisa Isaacson, MD*, Michael Babich, MD

KEYWORDS

• Hepatotoxicity • Drug-induced liver injury • Resources • Reporting

KEY POINTS

- To discuss the resources that are available to clinicians to aid in the diagnosis and management of drug-induced liver injury, including online databases and registries.
- To discuss how clinicians can report hepatotoxic drugs and view clinical trials available.

INTRODUCTION

Dr Hyman Zimmerman, a pioneer and major scholar of drug-induced liver injury (DILI), observed that a patient is at high risk of fatal DILI if consumption of a drug leads to hepatocellular injury in combination with jaundice as opposed to primarily cholestatic liver injury, better known as Hy's Law (**Box 1**).[1] His initial work in the later half of the twentieth century led to a comprehensive review of medications that were known to cause DILI, which are outlined in his original publication from 1978, *Hepatotoxicity: The Adverse Effects of Drugs and Other Chemicals on the Liver*.[2] However, it was not until 2013 that the first guidelines for the diagnosis and management of DILI were created by the Practice Parameters Committee of the American College of Gastroenterology.[3]

DILI has an estimated annual incidence between 1 per 10,000 to 100,000 persons exposed to prescription medications (most commonly antimicrobials and central nervous system agents) and is among the most common cause of acute liver failure (ALF) in the United States. It is the most common adverse indication leading to an individual drug's failure or withdrawal from the market.[4,5] Most new drugs are tested in fewer than 3000 people before approval; thus, DILI may not initially be detected. It is hypothesized that for every 10 cases of elevated alanine aminotransferase (ALT) >10 times the upper limit of normal (ULN) in a clinical trial, that there will be at least 1 case of

The authors have nothing to disclose.
Department of Gastroenterology and Hepatology, Allegheny General Hospital, 320 East North Avenue, Pittsburgh, PA 15212, USA
* Corresponding author.
E-mail address: marisa.isaacson@ahn.org

Clin Liver Dis 24 (2020) 131–139
https://doi.org/10.1016/j.cld.2019.09.010
1089-3261/20/© 2019 Elsevier Inc. All rights reserved.

liver.theclinics.com

> **Box 1**
> **Hy's law: 1 in 10 mortality risk in DILI provided the following 3 criteria are met**
>
> - Serum ALT or AST greater than 3 times ULN
> - Serum total bilirubin elevated to greater than 2 times ULN without initial findings of cholestasis (elevated Alk P)
> - The combination of increased aminotransferases and bilirubin cannot be explained by any other causes (eg, viral hepatitis A, B, C or other preexisting or acute liver disease)
>
> *Abbreviations:* Alk P, alkaline phosphatase; ALT, alanine aminotransferase; AST, aspartate aminotransferase; DILI, drug-induced liver injury; ULN, upper limit of normal.

severe liver injury that develops on widespread availability of that drug.[6] This, along with the plethora and consumption of unregulated dietary and herbal supplements, poses significant challenges with diagnosis and treatment of DILI. It has sparked widespread interest among clinicians (ranging from those in primary care, internal medicine, gastroenterology, toxicology), pharmaceutical companies, and regulatory bodies across the world, resulting in the creation of diagnostic scales, databases, registries, and reporting bodies to better understand DILI. The resources available are outlined and detailed in this article.

RESOURCES FOR THE CLINICIAN

The first step in the diagnosis of DILI is identifying possible culprits. A study published in 2015 assessed Food and Drug Administration (FDA)-approved drugs with reported hepatotoxicity, and noted that 49% (478 of 975 drugs examined) had the potential to induce adverse hepatic drug reactions based on their daily dose, liver metabolism, or lipophilicity.[7] Such a vast amount of hepatotoxic prescriptions, over-the-counter medications, and unregulated herbal and dietary supplements (HDSs) pose new challenges to the clinician in the assessment and management of DILI and has led to the advent of numerous registries and online hepatotoxicity resources for further guidance.[8,9]

LIVERTOX (https://livertox.nih.gov/resource.html)

Created in 2014 by the National Library of Medicine (NLM) and the Liver Disease Research Branch of the National Institute of Diabetes and Digestive and Kidney Diseases (NIDDK), LIVERTOX is a free Web site that provides concise, unbiased, accurate, and easily accessed drug records. It includes information on the details of hepatotoxicity caused by both prescription and nonprescription medications as well as HDSs. Drugs discussed include those that are currently approved or available in the United States. With a few exceptions, drugs withdrawn from the market, are no longer produced, or that are only available abroad are not addressed. In addition, topical creams and lotions, eye and ear drops, and nasal sprays are not included. As of 2018, LIVERTOX contained more than 1100 indexed agents and 23,000 annotated references. It is a dynamic resource and is updated periodically (every 2 to 3 years). To contribute to LIVERTOX, there is a Case Submission Registry through their interactive site, and participation in encouraged. All personal identifiers are removed and the submitted cases are maintained in a secure database for statistical analysis of trends in DILI and are linked to the individual drug records.[10]

UpToDate (https://www.uptodate.com)

UpToDate is an evidence-based clinician resource originally launched in 1992 by Dr Burton Rose. It initially began with topics in nephrology; however, it has vastly expanded to include more than 5200 articles across 25 different specialties. It includes a variety of medical and drug information and diagnostic scales. It is peer reviewed, and mandates the disclosure of conflict of interest by the authors of its articles. Although it does require an annual subscription fee, it is available through many medical institutions and offers continuing education/continuing medical education (CE/CME) credits.[11]

The Liver Toxicity Knowledge Base and the DILIrank Dataset (https://www.fda.gov/ScienceResearch/BioinformaticsTools/default.htm)

The Liver Toxicity Knowledge Base (LTKB), created by the FDA's National Center for Toxicologic Research scientists, compromises a benchmark dataset containing 287 FDA-approved drugs (which have been available for $\geq$10 years) with established potential to cause DILI based on the FDA-approved prescription drug label. Divided into 3 categories, these drugs are classified as most-DILI-concern (137 drugs), less-DILI-concern (85 drugs), and no-DILI-concern (65 drugs). The dataset summarizes the mechanisms of liver toxicity, histopathology, drug metabolism, therapeutic use, and side-effect profile.[12,13] An updated version, the DILIrank data set, at one time was the largest publicly available DILI data set containing 1036 FDA-approved drugs classified into 4 groups: 192 most-DILI-concern, 278 less-DILI-concern, 312 no-DILI-concern, 254 ambiguous-DILI-concern. The goals of the datasets are to improve the basic understanding of liver toxicity with the hope of developing predictive models and/or novel biomarkers, based on the knowledge accumulated from the early identification of DILI.[12]

Toxicogenomics Project-Genomic Assisted Toxicity Evaluation System (https://toxico.nibiohn.go.jp/english)

Toxicogenomics focuses on assessing the safety of compounds using their gene expression profiles and can be used to identify biomarkers for the evaluation and prediction of drug safety. The Toxicogenomics Project-Genomic Assisted Toxicity Evaluation System (Open TG-GATEs) is a large scale toxicogenomics database that stores gene expression profiles from both rat and human hepatocytes following exposure to 170 hepatotoxic and nephrotoxic compounds. Information available consists of biochemical, hematological, and histopathological data with digital pathologic images as well as gene expression data.[12,14,15]

Natural Medicines Comprehensive Database (https://naturalmedicines.therapeuticresearch.com)

The Natural Medicines Comprehensive Database is considered one of the most comprehensive and reliable natural medicine resources available and contains more than 1200 monographs on individual ingredients, providing evidence-based information on herbal and nonherbal supplements, natural medicines, and complementary and integrative therapy. It specifically addresses safety ratings, effectiveness ratings, and interaction ratings based on literature review. It is updated daily and undergoes rigorous peer review through a multipronged approach by health practitioners and appropriate content-area experts. Oftentimes, a newly discovered drug interaction or serious adverse event is added to the database within 24 hours. The database includes brand names, and allows the user to see which products contain specific hepatotoxic ingredients. It requires a subscription fee, and is available in a text version and as a phone application (app). CE/CME credit is available for health professionals when used online.[16,17]

Toxicology Data Network (https://toxnet.nlm.nih.gov)

The Toxicology Data Network (TOXNET) was created by the NLM in 1985 to provide more efficient access to an online group of databases. These databases contain toxicologic information regarding chemicals and other substances related to human exposure and their effect on our health. The included database TOXLINE, although not liver-specific, is useful in the search for hepatotoxic chemicals simply by typing phrases such as "liver toxicity," "hepatotoxicity," or "liver injury" into the search box. A single search results in an assortment of citations from multiple specialized journals (as well as nonspecialized sources such as PubMed and Medline) providing information on the biochemical, pharmacologic, physiologic, and toxicologic effects of various chemicals and drugs. It contains references dating as far back as the 1840s and is updated weekly.[18,19]

MedWatch (https://www.fda.gov/safety/medwatch)

Although DILI is the most common adverse event leading to drug failure during a clinical trial or withdrawal from the market, HDSs are not subjected to the same oversight process as are pharmaceuticals, and can be marketed without approval from the FDA.[9] The FDA monitors the reports of adverse events attributable to HDSs through its Center for Food Safety and Applied Nutrition and deems products unsafe when a question of toxicity arises. The Dietary Supplement Health Education and Safety Act of 1994 and the "Current Good Manufacturing Practice in Manufacturing, Packaging, Labeling, or Holding Operations for Dietary Supplements; Small Entity Compliance Guide of 2007" require the manufacturer to generate labels to market safe products and to report adverse events associated with their products.[20] The voluntary nature of adverse event reporting likely leads to underreporting; thus, consumers and clinicians are encouraged to use the reporting systems available, such as the Drug-Induced Liver Injury Network (DILIN) and MedWatch (discussed in the following paragraphs).[21]

MedWatch is a voluntary Web site used to report serious adverse events, product quality problems, medication error, therapeutic inequivalence, or drug failure that is suspected to be associated with the use of an FDA-regulated drug, a dietary supplement, or cosmetic. Counterfeit medical products can also be reported. Health care professionals and consumers are encouraged to visit the Web site to submit these events to keep effective products on the market and to ensure patient safety. After evaluation of the potential safety concern, the FDA may take regulatory action, such as restricting use of the drug, updating the labeling information, or even removing the drug from the market. These reports are kept in a database (FDA's Adverse Event Reporting System) and are available for those who wish to look for new safety concerns related to a product or to evaluate a manufacturer's compliance with reporting regulations.[22,23]

RESEARCH AND REGISTRIES

Given the idiosyncratic nature and low incidence of DILI, gaps in knowledge still remain despite advancements in medicine and the resources now available.

Drug-Induced Liver Injury Network (https://dilin.org)

The NIDDK has established the DILIN to conduct controlled clinical studies of DILI in attempts to close this knowledge gap. It is a consortium of 9 clinical centers across the

United States that collect and analyze cases of severe liver injury caused by prescription drugs, over-the-counter drugs, and alternative medicines (herbal products and supplements). Currently, both retrospective and prospective studies are being conducted.[24–33]

By initiating an ongoing prospective registry of patients with DILI, studies of host clinical, genetic, environmental, and immunologic risk factors can be performed and analyzed. Initially established in 2004, the prospective study consists of a nationwide registry of adults and children older than 2 years. Those who meet predefined eligibility criteria at their 6-month study visit are followed for 2 years with hopes to better understand the natural history of chronic DILI. Exclusion criteria, such as alternate established causes of liver disease, acetaminophen hepatotoxicity, or history of liver transplantation were established. Causality assessment is determined by the Roussel Uclaf Causality Assessment Method and "expert opinion," a panel of 3 expert hepatologists who independently assign a causality score as described previously. Once a minimum of 15 DILI cases due to a single medication are enrolled, up to 3 age-matched control subjects per case are identified to determine key differences in clinical risk factors. By establishing causality, the study strives to develop a repository of clinical data and biologic samples for further studies of DILI pathogenesis, genetic variability, and prevention.[4,34] As of 2017, the database contained more than 1200 patients with DILI caused by approximately 200 different agents.[8]

The retrospective study is also a nationwide registry; however, it includes those who have experienced liver injury within the past 10 years after consuming 1 of 8 drugs: phenytoin, isoniazid, amoxicillin/clavulanic acid, valproic acid, nitrofurantoin, trimethoprim-sulfamethoxazole, minocycline, and quinolone antibiotics. Goals of this study are not only to establish a database of patients with severe DILI due to any of the 8 aforementioned medications, but to also establish a bank of biological specimens from cases and controls, similar to the prospective study. Cases may be submitted to both the retrospective and prospective study through the DILIN Web site.[6] Numerous registries similar to the DILIN have also been formed globally, including in Australia, Spain, Iceland, India, and Korea.[35–39]

The Acute Liver Failure Study Group (https://www.utsouthwestern.edu/labs/acute-liver)

The Acute Liver Failure Study Group is a clinical research network initially established in 1997. Its mission is to gather important prospective data and biological samples from patients with ALF from any cause. It enrolls patients who meet the criteria for ALF (liver injury, abnormal coagulation testing, and abnormal mental functioning) at 13 different sites throughout North America. Since December 2016, more than 3000 patients have been enrolled in the registry. Not only have 2 phone apps been created (available through https://www.apple.com/ios/app-store), but multiple articles on various aspects of ALF have been published. Significant improvements in outcomes have been observed throughout the years that the study has been in operation.[40,41] Although the clinical characteristics, severity of the illness, and etiology of liver failure have not changed or declined, the number of patients requiring transplantation and those dying from ALF has decreased.[41]

Clinical Trials (https://clinicaltrials.gov)

The US FDA Modernization Act of 1997 amended the Federal Food, Drug, and Cosmetic Act with regulations to increase patient access to experimental drugs and medical devices, and to accelerate review of important new medications. These amendments included creation of the registry ClinicalTrials.gov, a database of clinical trials (both federally and privately supported) provided by the NLM. Currently, it lists more than 293,985 research studies being performed throughout the United States and 207 other countries throughout the world. It allows one to view a summary of the study protocol of interest, including the study description and design, the current status of the trial, and whether the trial is actively recruiting. Although not liver specific, it is simple to use, as one can enter their query into the search engine. It is available to both patients and researchers and is updated daily.[42,43]

CONFERENCES

Several conferences are held annually in efforts to update clinicians, exchange valuable information on patient care and research, and provide networking opportunities.

The Liver Meeting

Sponsored by the American Association for the Study of Liver Disease (AASLD), The Liver Meeting provides a forum for the exchange of the latest groundbreaking research in diseases of the liver and biliary tract, discussion of treatment options, and interaction with colleagues. The meeting is held annually, at various locations within the United States.[10,44] Worldwide, other meetings can be attended, such as the International Liver Congress organized by the European Association for the Study of the Liver and the Asian Pacific Association for the Study of the Liver annual meeting.[45,46]

The Drug-Induced Liver Injury Conference

The Drug-Induced Liver Injury Conference is cosponsored by the FDA, Center for Drug Evaluation and Research, and the Critical Path Institute and is endorsed by the National Institutes of Health, DILIN, AASLD, Hamner-UNC Institute for Drug Safety Sciences, and the Pharmaceutical Research and Manufacturers of America. This academic-industry-government conference is held annually, with presentations by experts in clinical hepatology and toxicology. It provides a forum to discuss new information and research on DILI, including ways to predict, measure, evaluate, and act on liver injury and dysfunction caused by medications (both in clinical trials and in post-marketing treatment groups).[10,47]

SUMMARY

Although many risk factors for developing DILI have been identified, and more than 1000 medications and HDSs are known to cause liver dysfunction, idiosyncratic drug reactions still remain unpredictable and erratic. Varying effects of individual drugs on the event cascade and patient genetic polymorphisms lead to different clinical presentations. Mechanisms and causality scales have been developed to guide the clinician in diagnosis, and several databases and registries are available for reference and reporting. Up-to-date information is regularly available to clinicians not only through frequent updating of these resources, but also through annual conferences that allow for networking and collaboration among colleagues. Our knowledge of DILI is far from complete, but it has come a long way since publication of the original studies and texts from the 1970s.

REFERENCES

1. Reuben A. Hy's law. Hepatology 2004;39(2):574–8.
2. Zimmerman HJ. Hepatotoxicity: the adverse effects of drugs and other chemicals on the liver. New York: Appleton-Century-Crofts; 1978.

3. Chalasani N, Hayashi P, Bonkovsky H, et al. Diagnosis and management of idiosyncratic drug-induced liver injury. Available at: https://gi.org/guideline/diagnosis-and-management-of-idiosyncratic-drug-induced-liver-injury. Accessed January 7, 2019.

4. Chalasani N, Fontana RJ, Bonkovsky HL, et al. Causes, clinical feature and outcomes from a prospective study of drug-induced liver injury in the United States. Gastroenterology 2008;135(6):1924.

5. Holt M, Ju C. Drug-induced liver injury. Handb Exp Pharmacol 2010;196:3–27.

6. Maddur H, Chalasani N. Idiosyncratic drug-induced liver injury: a clinical update. Curr Gastroenterol Rep 2011;13(1):65.

7. Wang Z, Wang K, Li H, et al. A comprehensive study of the association between drug hepatotoxicity and daily dose, liver metabolism and lipophilicity using 975 oral medications. Oncotarget 2015;6(19):17031–8.

8. Alempijevic T, Somon Z, Milosavijevic T. Drug induced liver injury: do we know everything? World J Hepatol 2017;9(10):491–502.

9. Available at: http://www.fda.gov/Food/DietarySupplements/default.htm. Accessed January 8, 2019.

10. National Institutes of Health. Available at: https://livertox.nih.gov/resource.html. Accessed January 6, 2019.

11. UpToDate®. Available at: http://www.uptodate.com. Accessed March 19, 2019.

12. Luo G, Shen Y, Yan L, et al. A review of drug-induced liver injury databases. Arch Toxicol 2017;91:3039–49.

13. National Center for Toxicological Research. Liver Toxicity Knowledge Base (LTKD). Available at: https://www.fda.gov/ScienceResearch/BioinformaticsTools/LiverToxicityKnowledgeBase/default.htm. Accessed January 9, 2019.

14. Igarash Y, Nakatsu N, Yamashita T. Open TG gates: a large-scale toxicogenomics database. Nucleic Acids Res 2015;43:D921–7.

15. Open TG-GATEs. Available at: https://toxico.nibiohn.go.jp/english. Accessed January 9, 2019.

16. Hsu PP. Natural medicines comprehensive database. J Med Libr Assoc 2002;90(1):114.

17. Natural Medicines Research Collaboration. Available at: https://naturalmedicines.therapeuticresearch.com. Accessed January 8, 2019.

18. U.S. National Library of Medicine. Available at: https://infocus.nlm.nih.gov. Accessed January 8, 2019.

19. TOXNET. Available at: https://toxnet.nlm.nih.gov. Accessed January 9, 2018.

20. Dietary supplements – guidance for industry: current good manufacturing practice in manufacturing, packaging, labeling or holding operations for dietary supplements; small entity compliance guide. Available at: https://www.fda.gov/food/guidanceregulation/guidancedocumentsregulatoryinformation/dietarysupplements/ucm238182.htm. Accessed January 10, 2019.

21. US Department of Health and Human Services Office of Inspector General. Adverse event reporting for dietary supplements: an inadequate safety valve. Washington, DC: AE Reporting; 2001.

22. Reporting serious problems to the FDA. Available at: https://www.fda.gov/safety/medwatch/howtoreport/default.htm. Accessed January 10, 2019.

23. FDA adverse event reporting system. Available at: https://www.fda.gov/drugs/guidancecomplianceregulatoryinformation/surveillance/adversedrugeffects. Accessed January 10, 2019.

24. DILIN. DILIN, online 2019. Available at: http://www.dilin.org. Accessed January 7,2019.

25. Suk KT, Kim DJ. Drug-induced liver injury: present and future. Clin Mol Hepatol 2012;18(3):249–57.
26. García-Cortés M, Stephens C, Lucena MI, et al. Causality assessment methods in drug induced liver injury: strengths and weaknesses. J Hepatol 2011;55: 683–91.
27. Benichou C, Danan G, Flahault A. Causality assessment of adverse reactions to drugs – II. An original model for validation of drug causality assessment methods: case reports with positive rechallenge. J Clin Epidemiol 1993; 46(11):1331–6.
28. Maria VA, Victorina RM. Development and validation of a clinical scale for the diagnosis of drug-induced hepatitis. Hepatology 1997;26(3):664–9.
29. Lucena MI, Camargo R, Andrade RJ, et al. Comparison of two clinical scales for causality assessment in hepatotoxicity. Hepatology 2001;33(1):123–30.
30. Naranjo CA, Busto U, Sellers EM, et al. A method for estimating the probability of adverse drug reactions. Clin Pharmacol Ther 1981;30:239–45.
31. Hayashi PH. Causality assessment in drug-induced liver injury. Semin Liver Dis 2009;29(4):348–56.
32. Lewis JH. Causality assessment: which is best, expert opinion or RUCAM? Hepatology. Available at: https://aasldpubs.onlinelibrary.wiley.com/doi/full/10.1002/cld365. Accessed January 7, 2019.
33. Rockey DC, Seeff LB, Rochon J, et al. Causality assessment in drug-induced liver injury using a structured expert opinion process: comparison to the Roussell-Uclaf causality assessment method. Hepatology 2010;51:2117–26.
34. Fontana R, Watkins P, Bnkovsky H. Drug-induced liver injury network (DILIN) prospective study. Drug Saf 2009;32(1):55–68.
35. Sistanizad M, Peterson GM. Drug-induced liver injury in the Australian setting. J Clin Pharm Ther 2013;38:115–20.
36. Andrade RJ, Lucena MI, Fernández MC, et al. Drug-induced liver injury: an analysis of 461 incidences submitted to the Spanish registry over a 10-year period. Gastroenterology 2005;129:512–21.
37. Björnsson ES, Bergmann OM, Björnsson HK, et al. Incidence, presentation, and outcomes in patients with drug-induced liver injury in the general population of Iceland. Gastroenterology 2013;144:1419–25.
38. Devarbhavi H, Dierkhising R, Kremers WK, et al. Single-center experience with drug-induced liver injury from India: causes, outcome, prognosis, and predictors of mortality. Am J Gastroenterol 2010;105:2396–404.
39. Suk KT, Kim DJ, Kim CH, et al. A prospective nationwide study of drug-induced liver injury in Korea. Am J Gastroenterol 2012;107(9):1380–7.
40. Acute Liver Failure Study Group. Available at: https://www.utsouthwestern.edu/labs/acute-liver/overview. Accessed January 9, 2019.
41. Reuben A, Tillman H, Fontana RJ, et al. Outcomes in adults with acute liver failure between 1998 and 2013: an observational cohort study. Ann Intern Med 2016; 164:724–32.
42. Clinical trials. Available at: http://www.clinicaltrials.gov. Accessed January 9, 2019.
43. Food and Drug Administration. Modernization act (FDAMA) of 1997. Available at: https://www.fda.gov/RegulatoryInformation/LawsEnforcedbyFDA/SignificantAmendmentstotheFDCAct/FDAMA/ucm089179.htm. Accessed January 9, 2019.
44. The liver meeting 2017. Available at: https://www.aasld.org/events-professional-development/liver-meeting. Accessed January 9, 2019.

45. European Association for the Study of the Liver. Available at: https://easl.eu. Accessed March 24, 2019.
46. Asian Pacific Association for the Study of the Liver. Available at: https://http://apasl.info. Accessed March 24, 2019.
47. Center for drug evaluation and research-DILI conference. Available at: https://www.fda.gov/Drugs/NewsEvents/ucm624334.htm. Accessed January 9, 2019.

Drug-induced Liver Injury Secondary to Herbal and Dietary Supplements

Elizabeth Zheng, MD[a], Naemat Sandhu, MD[b],
Victor Navarro, MD[b,*]

KEYWORDS

- Herbal and dietary supplement • Hepatoxicity • Liver injury

KEY POINTS

- The prevalence of hepatotoxicity attributable to herbal and dietary supplements is increasing in the US population and worldwide.
- Although herbal and dietary supplement–associated liver injury remains rare, its significance is marked by more severe liver injury and worse outcomes compared with drug-induced liver injury from conventional drug use.
- Given the multitude of potentially hepatotoxic ingredients in multi-ingredient supplements, the unknown concentrations, and possible mislabeling, as well as the largely undiscovered complexities of their interactions between substances and the host, the varying phenotypic presentation and spectrum of liver injury can be unpredictable, making the diagnosis challenging.
- Dietary supplements often contain green tea extract, which has been implicated as a hepatotoxic agent though positive rechallenge in human studies.

INTRODUCTION

The increasing usage of herbal and dietary supplements (HDS) and its significant impact on liver injury has been well documented.[1–4] The term HDS encompasses a wide range of ingredients, including vitamins, minerals, proteins, and herbs or other botanicals that have been used for purposes of supplementing a diet. In general, dietary supplements are commonly used to improve overall health and to enhance bodybuilding or weight loss efforts. Unlike conventionally prescribed medications, dietary supplements are under regulations of the 1994 Dietary Supplement Health and Education Act (DSHEA). Under this act, dietary supplements are not held to the same standards as prescription drugs and their efficacy as well as safety need not be proved before marketing.[5]

[a] Columbia University Medical Center, 622 West 168th Street, PH-14-406, New York, NY 10032, USA; [b] Einstein Medical Center, 5401 Old York Road, Klein Building Suite 505, Philadelphia, PA 19141, USA
* Corresponding author.
E-mail address: NavarroV@einstein.edu

Clin Liver Dis 24 (2020) 141–155
https://doi.org/10.1016/j.cld.2019.09.009
1089-3261/20/© 2019 Elsevier Inc. All rights reserved.
liver.theclinics.com

Although HDS-related hepatotoxicity is a concern, establishing direct causality of HDSs to liver injury is often a challenge because these supplements are usually composed of multiple ingredients and are prone to contamination or adulteration. The frequent mislabeling of HDSs poses an additional barrier in determining causality. Using 341 HDS samples collected from 1268 patients enrolled in the US Drug-Induced Liver Injury Network (DILIN), 203 products underwent chemical analysis and results were compared with the listed ingredients of product labels. Of the 203 products, only 90 (44%) HDSs had accurate labels reflecting the contents as determined by chemical analysis.[6]

This article reviews the impact of HDS-related liver injury in the United States and worldwide, explores the hepatotoxic potential of HDS products and ingredients, and highlights advancements in the use of toxicology in the study of HDS-related liver injury. In addition, as a result of the potential impact of HDS-related liver injury, there is a growing need for continued research and enhanced governmental regulations of HDS. This article therefore proposes future considerations for study with the goal of advancing knowledge and improving consumer safety.

HERBAL AND DIETARY SUPPLEMENT HEPATOTOXICITY IN THE UNITED STATES AND ABROAD

HDS usage has consistently increased over the past several decades, with recent estimates suggesting that up to one-half of the adult US population is taking dietary supplements.[3,7] Although proof of direct causality of hepatoxicity caused by HDSs is difficult to establish, the increasing recognition of drug-induced liver injury (DILI) from HDSs within the public domain and in the research community parallels the increasing rates of HDS usage. The DILIN has reported that the proportion of liver injury caused by HDSs has increased from 7% in 2004 to 2005 to 19% in 2010 to 2012, to 20% in 2013 to 2014.[4] As a result of these observations, it can reasonably be assumed that the prevalence of hepatotoxicity attributable to HDSs is increasing in the US population.

Although comprehensive population-based studies across the United States on DILI are lacking, attempts have been made to provide such estimates. In 2014, a prospective estimation of DILI was attempted in the state of Delaware. Gastroenterologists were asked to participate in surveillance for DILI and were able to identify 23 such patients in 2014. Of the 23 patients, 20 met DILIN criteria for suspected DILI, with 43% of cases being attributed to HDSs. Based on these data, the estimated incidence of DILI was 2.7 cases per 100,000 adults in 2014.[8] The study was the first prospective estimation of DILI in the United States, but incidence rates may be an underestimation because surveillance of DILI was limited to gastroenterologists. Although small in scale, this study underscores that events of liver injury caused by drugs and HDSs are rare.

Internationally, studies published in Spain and Iceland provide additional insight into the prevalence of DILI and HDS-related DILI. Among the few population-based studies, a survey of the Icelandic population revealed an incidence of DILI of 19.1 per 100,000 inhabitants per year. HDS-related liver injury comprised 16% of the cases, suggesting an approximate incidence of 3 per 100,000 persons.[9] A small population of primary doctors targeted through a robust system of outreach and recruitment may explain a higher prevalence than in the US study.

An increasing recognition of HDS-related liver injury has also occurred in Spain. On reviewing patients in the Spanish DILI registry from 1994 to 2004, only 2% of DILI cases were attributed to HDS. However, between 2010 and 2013, an increased rate of 13% was observed.[10] In addition to increasing rates of HDS-related hepatoxicity, the most recent data from the Spanish DILI registry have also suggested that HDS-induced liver injury is more severe than other types of DILI. From 1994 to 2016, 6% of patients with HDS-induced liver injury progressed to liver failure, compared with 4% of cases of conventional drugs, and no cases of anabolic androgenic–induced liver injury.[11]

Clinical Impact of Herbal and Dietary Supplement–associated Drug-induced Liver Injury

Although HDS-associated liver injury remains rare, its significance is marked by more severe liver injury and worse outcomes compared with DILI from conventional drug use. Based on results from a cohort of 1198 patients enrolled in the Acute Liver Failure Study Group (ALFSG), 133 (11.1%) were deemed by expert opinion to have DILI, with the most common cause being antimicrobials (46%). HDSs, nonprescription medications, and illicit substances were grouped under 1 category and responsible for 10.6% of cases. However, when this class was compared with antituberculosis drugs, there were fewer patients with spontaneous survival (21.4% vs 28%) and more required transplant (50% vs 40%). Similar results were observed compared with sulfur-containing drugs: patients who took HDSs, nonprescription medications, and illicit substances had worse spontaneous survival (21.4% vs 27.3%) and a higher proportion needed transplant (50% vs 36.4%).[12]

Using the same ALFSG database, Hillman and colleagues[13] examined the clinical features and outcomes of only patients with HDS-associated DILI from 1998 to 2015. Of note, previous nomenclature, as used in the 2016 publication, referred to HDSs as complementary and alternative medicines. However, the term HDS has now been largely adopted by the scientific community to describe this class of substances. The study's findings supported the increasing trend of HDS-associated liver injury, showing that HDS-associated DILI and liver failure increased between 1998 to 2007 and 2007 to 2015 (12.4% vs 21.1%). Notably, compared with patients with prescription medication DILI, the HDS population had a higher transplant rate (56% vs 32%) and lower rate of acute liver failure–specific 21-day transplant-free survival (17% vs 34%). Therefore, relative to DILI from antimicrobials or certain prescription medications, injury from HDS is rarer but should not be overlooked given its association with more severe injury leading to death or liver transplant.

COMMON CATEGORIES AND MULTI-INGREDIENT SUPPLEMENTS OF HERBAL AND DIETARY SUPPLEMENTS

Although HDSs encompass a multitude of products marketed for a variety of uses, they can be categorized into several main groups. These groups include bodybuilding products, such as anabolic steroids; multi-ingredient supplements for weight loss and energy enhancement; and herbal products, including traditional botanic products such as Chinese or Ayurvedic herbs.

Based on an interim analysis of the DILIN Prospective Study experience, there were 130 cases of liver injury caused by HDSs, of which at least 45 were attributed to bodybuilding supplements and the remaining 85 were attributed to 116 products, many of which contained multiple ingredients.[1] Similarly, in the Spanish DILI experience, most implicated HDS cases (60%) were induced by multi-ingredient products.[14] These studies highlight the consistent finding that multi-ingredient products have the potential to cause significant liver injury. Given the multitude of potentially hepatotoxic ingredients, the unknown concentrations, and possible mislabeling, as well as the largely undiscovered complexities of their interactions between substances and the host, the varying phenotypic presentation and spectrum of liver injury can be unpredictable. As such, it is important to recognize that diagnosing, determining causality, and prognosticating DILI caused by multi-ingredient substances can be challenging. The remainder of this article describes the most commonly used HDSs and classifies the phenotypic characteristics of liver injury attributed to products or ingredients that have been implicated as causes of hepatotoxicity (Table 1).

ANABOLIC ANDROGENIC STEROIDS

Anabolic androgenic steroids (AASs) are typically marketed as bodybuilding supplements. AAS are synthetic derivatives of testosterone and are mainly indicated for treatment of male hypogonadism, hereditary angioneurotic edema, breast cancer, and anemia.[15] Synthetic AAS were developed with the intent to have preferential anabolic activity for increased performance enhancement and muscle building rather than their androgenic or masculinizing properties.[16]

A 2014 meta-analysis of 187 studies showed a lifetime prevalence of AAS use of 6.4% for men and 1.6% for women.[17] However, the use of AAS has increased in the last 2 decades. With regard to bodybuilding HDS cases, the DILIN has reported an increase from 2% in 2004 to 2005 to 8% in 2010 to 2012. Bodybuilding products were the most common cause for liver injury in those using HDS products.[1] Similarly, the Spanish DILI registry noted an increase from 1% in 1994 to 2009 to 8% in 2010 to 2013 for cases of AAS-induced hepatotoxicity.[11] This uptrend in prevalence worldwide is likely a combination of increased usage of AAS and improved clinical awareness of this form of liver injury.

Since the discovery of testosterone in the 1930s, synthetic derivatives that are orally active and possess prolonged biological activity have been produced. Derivatives made by 17-alpha-alkylation, such as methyltestosterone, methandrostenolone, oxymetholone, oxandrolone, and stanozol, are resistant to inactivation through first-pass hepatic metabolism, making them potentially hepatotoxic.[16] With increasing use of AASs in the general population, AASs are designed to closely resemble the original active compounds but with enough chemical diversity that ensures difficult detection during chemical analysis.[18] Many of these so-called designer AASs are available as over-the-counter dietary or bodybuilding supplements. A few commonly known designer steroids in dietary supplements are methasterone, prostanozol, androstatrienedione, epiandrosterone, blodenone, and dimethazine.

The most distinct phenotypic form of liver injury is characterized by prolonged and intense cholestasis.[19–21] This clinical picture is typically a young man using an HDS for the purposes of increasing muscle mass or performance enhancement. The injury typically occurs within 1 to 4 months of initiating AAS use. On presentation, there is jaundice caused by increased total bilirubin levels up to 40 to 50 mg/dL, and this is usually accompanied by a modest increase of transaminase levels with minimal to no increase in alkaline phosphatase level. On histology, this form of liver injury is referred to as bland cholestasis, as shown by marked canalicular cholestasis with minimal portal inflammation and necrosis.[1,4,11,19]

Jaundice from AAS and bodybuilding HDS can last up to 3 months and is generally associated with nonfatal outcomes, unlike other HDSs, such as nonbodybuilding multi-ingredient supplements. In the DILIN study, no cases of liver injury from a bodybuilding HDS required liver transplant, compared with 13% of cases from nonbodybuilding HDSs and 3% of cases from conventional medications. No fatalities were noted in the bodybuilding HDS group, as opposed to 7% and 3% mortality with

Table 1
Phenotypes and unique characteristics of commonly encountered multi-ingredient supplements

Supplement	Marketed Uses	Suspected Hepatotoxic Agents	Predominant Pattern of Liver Injury	Comments
AAS	Bodybuilding, Performance enhancement	C-17 alkylated testosterones	Acute cholestasis (common), Hepatocellular	• Bland cholestasis is characteristic of AAS hepatotoxicity. • Renal dysfunction can be concurrent with cholestasis. • Generally nonfatal outcomes
OxyELITE Pro	Weight loss, Bodybuilding, Fat burning, Performance enhancement	Aegeline	Hepatocellular	• Reported cases of acute hepatitis with confluent, submassive, or massive necrosis requiring liver transplant • Can be associated with autoimmune features requiring immune suppressive therapy • Mortality of 10% in cases of jaundice[61] • Hepatotoxicity may be associated with newer formulations containing Aegeline
SLIMQUICK	Weight loss	Green tea extract (Camellia sinensis)	Hepatocellular	• Mild to moderate injury, but has caused severe hepatocellular injury requiring liver transplant[62]
Move Free	Joint health	Chinese skullcap (Scutellaria baicalensis), Black catechu (Acacia catechu), Uniflex (mineral complex)	Hepatocellular	• Self-limited, mild to moderate severity of injury • One case of positive rechallenge[63]
Herbalife	Weight loss, Digestive health, General health and well-being, Boosting energy and immunity	Green tea extract (C sinensis), Gingko, Saw palmetto	Hepatocellular (common), Mixed	• Acute hepatitis with cholestatic features on biopsy • Prolonged latency period until onset of injury. Up to 2–9 mo after initiation of Herbalife supplement • Positive rechallenge reported[64]
Hydroxycut	Weight loss, Bodybuilding, Fat burning	Ephedra, Green tea extract (C sinensis), Aloe vera extract	Hepatocellular	• Acute self-limited viral hepatitis–like syndrome • Fatal cases resulting in death or liver transplant • Most presenting with jaundice[65]

Abbreviation: AAS, anabolic androgenic steroids.

conventional medications and nonbodybuilding HDS groups, respectively.[1] Several cases have had accompanying renal dysfunction, occasionally requiring transient renal replacement therapy, but both liver and renal injury ultimately have been noted to resolve.[4,19,20] Cholestatic injury usually reverts after discontinuation of AAS.[22]

The pattern of cholestatic hepatitis from AAS suggests that there is selective impairment of biliary canalicular function that may be caused by inhibition or dysfunction of biliary transporter proteins such as ATPase phospholipid transporting 8B1 (ATP8B1) and ATP binding cassette subfamily B member 11 (ABCB11). Such impairment can lead to disruption of bilirubin or bile acid transport and secretion.[23]

Vascular changes in the liver, referred to as peliosis hepatis, have also been linked to prolonged use of oral anabolic steroids. This condition is a rare syndrome characterized by enlarged blood-filled sinusoids and loss of endothelial barriers. Typically, peliosis hepatis is seen among patients with advanced wasting diseases, tuberculosis, and cancer. However, peliosis associated with anabolic steroids usually reverses, at least to some degree, with discontinuation of the therapy.[16]

One of the most serious complications from anabolic steroid use is the development of benign or malignant hepatic neoplasms such as adenomas or hepatocellular carcinoma. They usually occur after prolonged use of androgenic steroids, such as in cases of hypogonadism or aplastic anemia in which steroids have been used for 2 to 4 years. However, there have been occasional cases observed among patients who have used AASs for bodybuilding without underlying liver disease. Compared with oral contraceptive–associated hepatic adenomas, the cases of anabolic steroid-induced hepatic adenoma are rare. Cases reported have shown regression of the adenomas over a period of 6 months to 1 year with near to complete resolution after withdrawal of the offending anabolic steroid.[16,24]

DIETARY SUPPLEMENTS FOR WEIGHT LOSS AND OBESITY IN THE UNITED STATES

Obesity rates have been increasing in the United States over the past several decades, with its prevalence reported as high as 35% among men and 40.4% among women in 2013 to 2014.[25] The increase in obesity rates has been accompanied by the popularity of dietary supplements marketed for weight loss, with an estimated 15.2% of US adults ever having used a weight loss supplement.[26] In a survey of 3500 US adults who made a serious weight loss attempt, 33.9% reported using a dietary supplement.[27] Therefore, it was not surprising when the DILIN study reported that, from 2004 to 2013, dietary supplements for the purpose of weight loss were among the most common products within the nonbodybuilding HDS category.[1] This article defines weight loss products as dietary supplements that have been marketed for the purposes of weight loss/reduction, fat burning, or metabolism boosting.

Popular weight loss products such as Hydroxycut and OxyELITE Pro (OEP) have been reported to cause a hepatocellular pattern of liver injury with significant morbidity requiring liver transplant.[28,29] Although the relation to increased severity of liver injury is unknown, it should be recognized that these are multi-ingredient supplements and therefore carry an additional layer of complexity with regard to host effects, interactions among all the ingredients, and potential of product mislabeling. Despite the multitude of substances used in 1 weight loss product, the possible hepatotoxic culprits that have received research attention include green tea extract (GTE) and *Garcinia cambogia* extract. The toxicity of these specific ingredients is discussed in further detail later.

In the spring and summer of 2013, an outbreak of acute hepatitis and liver failure occurred in Hawaii among 7 patients with a history of OEP usage for the intent of weight loss or muscle building. Their experience and outcomes have previously been described.[30] By September 2013, the Hawaii Department of Health was notified of the individuals who had all been exposed to OEP. As a result, physicians were notified to report any known cases of adults who had used any product labeled OEP for weight loss or muscle building before illness onset.

Subsequently, a retrospective review was conducted on any known cases as defined by individuals with acute-onset hepatitis of unknown cause on or after April 1 2013, a history of weight loss/muscle building dietary supplement use during the 60 days before illness onset, and residence in Hawaii during the period of exposure. The study revealed a total of 76 reports, 44 (58%) of which met the case definition, with 41 probable cases and 3 suspected cases. Of the 41 probable cases, 34 reported OEP exposure, although 7 patients were also exposed to another supplement. Among this cohort of patients, 2 required liver transplant and 1 died.[31] Although the pattern of injury was largely hepatocellular, all OEP-exposed patients reported having dark urine and 92% reported jaundice, fatigue, and decreased appetite.

On review of OEP product formulation from January to September 2013, there were 2 commercially available types of OEP: a 1,3-demthylamylamine (DMAA)–containing OEP, which was the original formula, and multiple DMAA-free OEP formulations that became available in late 2012. Most reported patients (83%) used at least 1 DMAA-free formulation. This type of formulation contained an additional ingredient, aegeline, a plant-derived substance that has been used in Ayurvedic medicine. However, the hepatotoxic potential of aegeline and other ingredients in OEP remains unknown and further research is required to determine the truly implicated substances.

Similar results were found in the DILIN database from May to December 2013. Liver injury attributed to OEP was observed in 6 cases (5 women) and all presented with a hepatocellular pattern of injury.[32] There were 2 patients who required liver transplant.

Before the reported cases of OEP-induced liver injury, another popular weight loss product, called Hydroxycut, also garnered attention from the medical community. In 2009, the US Food and Drug Administration (FDA) issued a warning about supplements sold under the Hydroxycut label after 23 cases of liver injury were attributed to the product. In one of the largest case series, describing 8 patients with liver injury associated with Hydroxycut, all had a hepatocellular pattern of injury, with 5 spontaneous recoveries and 3 requiring liver transplant.[33] Similar to OEP and inherent to the nature of multi-ingredient HDS-induced liver injury, the hepatotoxic ingredients remain unknown. However, several specific ingredients that are commonly used in multi-ingredient supplements have been shown to have hepatotoxic potential. These individual ingredients are reviewed next (**Table 2**).

SUSPECTED TOXIC INGREDIENTS IN MULTI-INGREDIENT SUPPLEMENTS
Green Tea Extract

GTE is a substance derived from the Chinese tea tree, *Camellia sinensis*, and is composed of catechins and polyphenolic flavanols. The most abundant catechin, epigallocatechin gallate (EGCG), is thought to be the active ingredient of GTE. Given the alleged antiobesity properties of EGCG by the inhibition of lipogenic enzymes, GTE is frequently included in multi-ingredient dietary supplements to promote weight loss.[34] Despite the possible weight loss benefits, GTE has been shown to cause liver injury through mitochondrial damage and formation of reactive oxygen species, thus inducing oxidative stress and hepatocellular apoptosis.[35,36]

A threshold dose has been observed in mice models in which a single dose of 1500 mg/kg of EGCG causes significant increase in alanine transaminase (ALT) level and increase in mortality. The results were similar when mice were given the same

Table 2
Suspected individual hepatotoxic ingredients

Hepatotoxic Ingredient	Marketed Use	Mechanism of Injury	Comments
Green Tea Extract (*C sinensis*)	Weight loss	Mitochondrial damage and oxidative stress	Hepatotoxicity may be dose dependent and more likely to occur in the fasting state
G cambogia	Weight loss	Oxidative stress	Associated with hepatic fibrosis and inflammation
Usnic acid (*Usnea* lichens)	Weight loss	Mitochondrial dysfunction and oxidative stress	Has a broad spectrum of biological attributes, including antimicrobial, antiviral, and antiinflammatory properties but potential for hepatotoxicity limits its use
Ephedra/ma huang (*Ephedra sinica*)	Weight loss	Mitochondrial damage and oxidative stress	The active component has the same properties of ephedrine and pseudoephedrine
Kava (*Piper methysticum*)	Anxiolytic, sedation, relaxation	Mitochondrial damage	Liver injury can be severe, leading to fulminant liver failure
Kratom (*Mitragyna* species)	Analgesic, stimulant, opioid withdrawal	Unknown	Pattern of liver injury is primarily cholestatic

dose but split into 2 days (750 mg/kg/d). However, when the dosage was reduced to 500 mg/kg/d, less hepatotoxicity was observed, suggesting a threshold total daily dose.[37] The estimated equivalent doses of EGCG in humans were 30 to 90 mg/kg, which is equivalent to 10 to 32 cups of green tea daily. The documented amount of EGCG in weight loss products is less than this suggested threshold dose, but, without performing toxicology on each product, the true amount of EGCG remains unknown.

Convincing clinical data on the potential hepatotoxic effect of GTE on human liver come from the Minnesota Green Tea Trial, in which healthy postmenopausal women with no chronic liver disease were given GTE to be taken twice daily for 12 months (total daily tea catechins of 1315 mg, including 843 mg of EGCG, which is the equivalent of approximately 5 cups of 235 mL [8 oz] brewed green tea per day).[38] The purpose of the study was to assess the effect of daily GTE consumption on biomarkers of breast cancer risk among patients. Women were randomized to either the GTE group or placebo group. On detailed analysis, 8.6% of women who received GTE developed an increased ALT level more than 1.25 times the upper limit of normal (ULN), compared with 1.8% of women in the placebo arm. In addition, 3.3% of women who had taken GTE developed moderate or severe increases in liver enzyme levels (ALT>2.5 × ULN), whereas no women developed moderate or severe increases in liver enzyme levels in the placebo group. There were no statistically significant differences in baseline characteristics such as age, race, education, body mass index, use of alcohol, history of smoking, use of aspirin, other nonsteroidal antiinflammatory drugs or acetaminophen, and use of statin. ALT levels returned to less than 90 U/L after a mean of 32 days of GTE discontinuation in all women.

Although the study did not establish a threshold dose effect of EGCG on liver injury, it did confirm the association of liver injury with high-dose EGCG consumption, particularly when liver injury was again observed in instances of GTE resumption. Among women who experienced liver injury the first time they were exposed to GTE, more than half who took GTE a second time, and all the women who took GTE a third time, experienced an increased ALT level more than 1.5 times ULN. This rechallenge phenomenon serves as vital evidence for the casual relationship between GTE and hepatotoxicity. However, further investigation is needed to determine the threshold dose effect in humans and to elucidate why a certain minority of patients are more susceptible to liver injury from EGCG compared with others.

Garcinia cambogia

G cambogia, also known as the Malabar tamarind, is a fruit commonly grown in Asia. The rind of the fruit contains the active ingredient hydroxycitric acid and has been found to have the ability to inhibit the conversion of carbohydrates to fat in vivo.[39] In mice models, G cambogia altered adipogenesis and ameliorated visceral adiposity.[40] Not surprisingly, this ingredient is commonly found in weight loss products such as Hydroxycut, Herbalife, and Fruta Planta Life. As stated elsewhere in this article, Hydroxycut has been associated with cases of liver injury, although direct injury caused by G cambogia cannot be established given the multitude of other ingredients. Laboratory studies have shown an association with hepatic fibrosis, inflammation, and oxidative stress.[41]

Usnic Acid

Also used in dietary supplements, usnic acid is a naturally occurring compound found in several different lichen species. It has a broad spectrum of biological attributes, including antimicrobial, antiviral, and antiinflammatory properties.[42–44] Despite its useful activities, it has also been known to cause hepatotoxicity, although the precise mechanism needs further elucidation. Prior studies have suggested toxicity from oxidative stress and disruption of mitochondrial function.[45,46]

Ephedra

The herb Ephedra sinica, also known as Chinese ephedra or ma huang, contains alkaloid compounds that have the same effect as ephedrine and pseudoephedrine. Although it may be a cardiovascular stimulant, studies have also reported its association with liver injury. The exact mechanism of hepatotoxicity requires further investigation, although in vitro studies have shown mitochondrial oxidative stress in ephedrine-treated hepatic stellate cells.[47]

Kava Kava

The kava root, Piper methysticum, is a plant indigenous to the Hawaiian, Polynesian, and Fiji islands and is a traditional medicinal product used for its anxiolytic properties. The first confirmed case of kava-induced liver injury was reported in 1998 because of a positive reexposure test.[48] Degrees of hepatotoxicity caused by kava ranging from cholestatic hepatitis to fulminant liver failure requiring liver transplant have been documented in a previous case series.[49] Although data from in vivo studies are lacking, in vitro studies have shown cell apoptosis likely caused by mitochondrial dysfunction when exposed to a kava alkaloid, pipermethystine.[50]

Kratom

Commonly known as kratom, the plant *Mitragyna* species is indigenous to southeast Asia and its leaves have been used in traditional medicines for its opioid, analgesic, and stimulantlike properties. Over the past several years, kratom use in the form of tea, capsules, or leaves for smoking or chewing has gained popularity in the Western world for managing fatigue and chronic pain, as well as treating opioid withdrawal.[51] Recently, liver injury caused by kratom use has been documented in rare case reports. The pattern of liver injury seems to be largely cholestatic and the cause of hepatoxicity requires further research.[52,53]

TOXICOLOGY IN HERBAL AND DIETARY SUPPLEMENTS

Establishing the diagnosis of liver injury and attributing causality to HDSs is challenging. It requires a stepwise process of eliminating alternative causes that can have a similar presentation. The use of toxicology and chemical analysis to aid in the diagnosis of DILI caused by HDSs by determining the culprit hepatotoxic ingredient can be promising. However, assessment of HDS toxicity poses its own challenges, because products frequently contain multiple ingredients with unclear chemical descriptors. These chemical descriptors are a symbolic representation of a molecule on analysis, which can be based on the constitution, topography, and molecular properties. The analysis of descriptors and their individual significance can be an exhaustive process. Based on a 2013 study from China, for each herbal compound, 1664 descriptors were calculated. However, after exclusion of redundant descriptors, only 135 remained.[54] There can also be contamination with microbials, pharmaceuticals, heavy metals, and mycotoxins.[55,56] In addition, large batch-to-batch variations in the content of the completed HDS product can exist.[57] Conventional toxicologic analysis involves both in vitro and in vivo testing of a component to determine cellular and organ toxicity.

The DILIN has recently used toxicologic analysis of HDSs to confirm the suspicion that multi-ingredient supplements can contain more components than advertised. The analysis confirmed the presence of ingredients that were not listed on individual labels of the HDSs. The rate of mislabeling of the supplements was up to 48% to 80%, the highest being for bodybuilding and weight loss products.[6] This finding confirms the complexity of ingredients among HDSs, which may be a factor in its association with severe liver injury. In the future, with the use of toxicologic analysis, products implicated in DILI can be interrogated and their component parts subjected to further toxicologic analysis.

Future research endeavors will add more to the knowledge regarding the toxicity of HDSs. The National Toxicology Program and Botanical Supplements Program have advanced technology in chromatography and mass spectrometry to aid in the determination of the chemical and physical composition of suspected harmful HDSs. In addition, The Office of Dietary Supplements has been established by the National Institutes of Health (NIH) to create a knowledge base and is given resources to conduct or support research on specific supplements. This broad mandate promotes the development of a comprehensive database regarding the potential toxicity of ingredients within the HDS products.[58]

FUTURE CONSIDERATIONS

The long-standing law that protects supplement manufacturers does not provide adequate protection to the consumer, allowing consumers to be exposed to products that have hepatotoxic potential. Therefore, it is incumbent on the scientific community to document and investigate each instance of liver injury attributed to an HDS. DILI caused by an HDS may be the result of a limited, albeit complex number of factors centered around host characteristics and hepatotoxic agents. Viewed in this way, a research agenda that ultimately results in a standard guideline for consumers and manufacturers can be designed to promote a safer supplement market while working within the framework of the existing law **(Fig. 1)**.

First, injury can result from products that are inherently toxic. Such toxicity can be dose related, as in the case of GTE in animals, or idiosyncratic. Dose-dependent toxic agents should be documented such that supplement manufacturers are not prohibited from their use but limited in their quantity to ensure that the threshold dose of toxicity cannot be reached. Consumers should also be made aware that overuse of a product can result in hepatotoxicity.

Second, injury may result not only from overuse but also misuse. For example, weight loss products containing GTE can be used in circumstances that may enhance their toxicity, such as during periods of extreme exercise or dehydration and inanition.[59] Thus, these circumstances should be recorded to guide consumers on how to safely consume these products. Third, there may be genetic predisposition to injury, as suggested in a recent study investigating genetic variants among patients with idiosyncratic DILI.[60] In a genome-wide association study among patients with idiosyncratic DILI, a polymorphism found on the gene PTPN22 was associated with an increased risk of liver injury caused by multiple drugs, particularly with amoxicillin and clavulanate. These promising findings highlight the future technological advances in the study of DILI. Although the genetic basis is likely to be unknown to most consumers in the near future, the continued study and discovery of genetic predisposition will be helpful in aiding future diagnoses of DILI.

As previously mentioned, HDS products are not subject to the same FDA drug regulations as prescription medications and are not mandated to undergo investigational clinical trials. Therefore, reporting of postmarketing adverse events largely depends on clinicians. However, the systems for reporting adverse reactions remain voluntary and passive. As a result, the reports can be fragmented, not standardized, and of

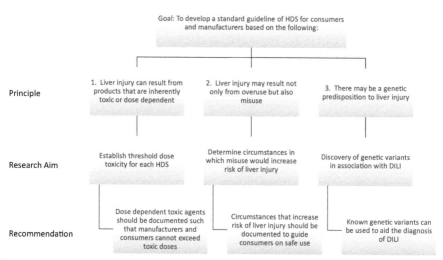

Fig. 1. Future considerations in the study of liver injury caused by HDS.

uneven quality.[58] Hence, failing any headway in scientific progress to improve the safety of HDSs, a more robust approach to clinician reporting and regulatory enforcement may improve consumer safety.

SUMMARY

HDS-associated DILI has now been well documented and, with increasing global use and recognition, the prevalence has been increasing. The variety of products, complexity of multi-ingredient supplements, and unknown concentrations, as well as additional unlabeled substances, have made the diagnosis and prognostication of DILI challenging, necessitating further research and attention by the scientific community. Broad categories of HDSs described in this article include, but are not limited to, AAS, multi-ingredient supplements for weight loss, and popular individual ingredients with documented hepatotoxic potential.

Despite such a large array of products and an increasing prevalence, HDS-associated liver injury still comprises a minority of cases compared with DILI induced by prescription medications or antimicrobials. However, the significance of DILI from HDS consumption deserves special attention because liver injury has been shown to cause more severe outcomes, thus more frequently necessitating liver transplant. In addition, although this article summarizes characteristics of both multi-ingredient supplements and individual agents, the former seems to cause more concern with regard to severity of liver injury, as documented, for example, in weight loss supplements such as Hydroxycut and OEP. The potential for more severe liver injury among these products remains unknown and may be in the setting of complex interactions between individual ingredients, supplement overuse, or combination use with other drugs.

Although the scientific community has already made great progress in investigating HDS-associated DILI through documentation, use of toxicology, and in vitro studies, continued vigilance in diagnosing DILI caused by HDSs and ongoing research are essential for improving consumer safety. As further exploration in this topic yields greater scientific evidence, it is hoped that these advances will be used as the foundation for improved regulatory enforcement and guidance for consumers to aid in safe consumption.

REFERENCES

1. Navarro V, Barnhart H, Bonkovsky HL, et al. Liver injury from herbals and dietary supplements in the U.S. drug induced liver injury network. Hepatology 2014; 60(4):1399–408.

2. Zhou Y, Yang L, Liao Z, et al. Epidemiology of drug induced liver injury in China; a systematic analysis of the Chinese literature including 21,789 patients. Eur J Gastroenterol Hepatol 2013;25(7):825–9.

3. Bailey RL, Gahche JJ, Lentino CV, et al. Dietary supplement use in the United States, 2003-2006. J Nutr 2011;141:261–6.

4. Navarro VJ, Khan I, Bjornsson E, et al. Liver injury from herbal and dietary supplements. Hepatology 2017;65(1):363–73.

5. Food and Drug Administration. Dietary Supplements. 2016. Available at: http://www.fda.gov/Food/DietarySupplements/default.htm. Accessed February 20, 2016.

6. Navarro V, Khan I, Avula B, et al. The frequency of herbal and dietary supplement mislabeling: experience of the drug induced liver injury network. Hepatol Commun 2017. https://doi.org/10.1002/hep.29501.

7. Clarke TC, Black LI, Stussman BJ, et al. National Health Statistics reports: no 79. Hyattsville (MD): National Center for Health Statistics; 2015. Trends in the use of complementary health approaches among adults: United States, 2002–2012.

8. Vega M, Verma M, Beswick D, et al. The incidence of drug and herbal and dietary supplement induced liver injury: preliminary findings from gastroenterologist based surveillance in the population of the state of Delaware. Drug Saf 2017; 40(9):783–7.

9. Bjornsson ES, Bergmann OM, Bjornsson HK, et al. Incidence, presentation, and outcomes in patients with drug-induced liver injury in the general population of Iceland. Gastroenterology 2013;144(7):1419–25, 1425.e1–3. [quiz: e19–20].

10. Andrade RJ, Lucena MI, Fernández MC, et al. Spanish group for the study of drug-induced liver disease. Gastroenterology 2005;129(2):512–21.

11. Robles-Diaz M, Gonzalez-Jimenez A, Medina-Caliz I, et al, Spanish DILI Registry, LatinDILI Network. Distinct phenotype of hepatotoxicity associated with illicit use of anabolic androgenic steroids. Aliment Pharmacol Ther 2015;41(1):116–25.

12. Reuben A, Koch D, Lee W, et al. Drug-induced acute liver failure: results of a U.S. Multicenter prospective study. Hepatology 2010;52(6):2065–76.

13. Hillman L, Gottfried M, Whitsett M, et al. Clinical features and outcomes of complementary and alternative medicine induced acute liver failure and injury. Am J Gastroenterol 2016;111(7):958–65.

14. Medina-Caliz I, Garcia-Cortes M, Gonzalez-Jimenez A, et al. Herbal and dietary supplement-induced liver injuries in the Spanish DILI registry. Clin Gastroenterol Hepatol 2018;16(9):1495–502.

15. Smith DA, Perry PJ. The efficacy of ergogenic agents in athletic competition Part I: androgenic-anabolic steroids. Ann Pharmacother 1992;26:520–8.

16. Solimini R, Rotolo MC, Mastrobattista L, et al. Hepatotoxicity associated with illicit use of anabolic androgenic steroids in doping. Eur Rev Med Pharmacol Sci 2017; 21(1 Suppl):7–16.

17. Sagoe D, Molde H, Andreassen CS, et al. The global epidemiology of anabolic-androgenic steroid use: a meta-analysis and meta-regression analysis. Ann Epidemiol 2014;24(5):383–98.

18. Rahnema CD, Crosnoe LE, Kim ED. Designer steroids- over-the-counter supplements and their androgenic component: review of an increasing problem. Andrology 2015;3(2):150–5.

19. Krishnan PV, Feng ZZ, Gordon SC. Prolonged intrahepatic cholestasis and renal failure secondary to anabolic androgenic steroid-enriched dietary supplements. J Clin Gastroenterol 2010;43:672–5.

20. Kafrouni MI, Anders RA, Verma S. Hepatotoxicity associated with dietary supplements containing anabolic steroids. Clin Gastroenterol Hepatol 2007;5:809–12.

21. Cabb E, Baltar S, Powers DW, et al. The diagnosis and manifestation of liver injury secondary to off-label androgenic anabolic steroid use. Case Rep Gastroenterol 2016;10:499–505.

22. Shahidi NT. A review of the chemistry, biologic action, and clinical applications of anabolic-androgenic steroids. Clin Ther 2001;23(9):1355–90.

23. El Sherif Y, Potts JR, Howard MR, et al. Hepatotoxicity from anabolic androgenic steroids marketed as dietary supplements: contribution from ATP8B1/ABCB11 mutations? Liver Int 2013;33:1266–70.

24. Socas L, Zumbado M, Perez-Luzardo, et al. Hepatocellular adenomas associated with anabolic androgenic steroid abuse in bodybuilders: a report of two cases and a review of the literature. Br J Sports Med 2005;39(5):e27.

25. Flegal KM, Kruszon-Moran D, Carroll MD, et al. Trends in obesity among adults in the United States, 2005 to 2014. JAMA 2016;315(21):2284–91.

26. Blacnk HM, Serdula MK, Gillespie C, et al. Use of nonprescription dietary supplements for weight loss is common among Americans. J Am Diet Assoc 2007; 107(3):441–7.

27. Pillitteri JL, Shiffman S, Rohay JM, et al. Use of dietary supplements for weight loss in the United States: results of a national survey. Obesity 2008;16(4):790–6.

28. Roytman MM, Psrzgen P, Lee CL, et al. Outbreak of severe hepatitis linked to weight loss supplement OxyELITE Pro. Am J Gastroenterol 2014;109:1296–8.

29. Fong TL, Klontz KC, Canas-Coto A, et al. Hepatotoxicity due to Hydroxycut: a case series. Am J Gastroenterol 2010;105:1561–6.

30. Centers for Disease Control and Prevention (CDC). Notes from the field: acute hepatitis and liver failure following the use of a dietary supplement intended for weight loss or muscle building. MMWR Morb Mortal Wkly Rep 2013;62:817–9.

31. Johnston DI, Chang A, Viray M, et al. Hepatotoxicity associated with the dietary supplement OxyELITE Pro – Hawaii, 2013. Drug Test Anal 2016;8(3–4):319–27.

32. Heidemann LA, Navarro VJ, Ahmad J, et al. Erratum to: severe acute hepatocellular injury attributed to OxyELITE Pro: a case series. Dig Dis Sci 2016;61(12): 3638.

33. Kaswala D, Shah S, Patel N, et al. Hydroxycut-induced liver toxicity. Ann Med Health Sci Res 2014;4(1):143–5.

34. Wolfram S, Wang Y, Thielecke F. Anti-obesity effects of green tea: from bedside to bench. Mol Nutr Food Res 2006;50:176–87.

35. Moon HS, Lee HG, Choi YJ, et al. Proposed mechanisms of epigallocatechin-3-gallate for anti-obesity. Chem Biol Interact 2007;167(2):85–98.

36. Galati G, Lin A, Sultan A, et al. Cellular and in vivo hepatotoxicity caused by green tea phenolic acids and catechins. Free Radic Biol Med 2006;40(4):570–80.

37. Lambert JD, Kennett MJ, Sang S, et al. Hepatotoxicity of high oral dose (−)-epigallocatechin-3-gallate in mice. Food Chem Toxicol 2010;48(1):409–16.

38. Yu Z, Hamed S, Dostal A, et al. Effect of green tea supplements on liver enzyme elevation: results from a randomized intervention study in the United States. Cancer Prev Res (Phila) 2017;10(10):571–9.

39. Triscari J, Sullivan AC. Comparative effects of (-)-hydroxycitrate and (+)-allohydroxycitrate on acetyl CoA carboxylase and fatty acid and cholesterol synthesis in vivo. Lipids 1977;12:357–63.

40. Kim KY, Lee HN, Kim YJ, et al. Garcinia cambogia extract ameliorates visceral adiposity in C57BL/6K mice fed on a high-fat diet. Biosci Biotechnol Biochem 2008;72:1772–80.

41. Kim YJ, Choi MS, Park YB, et al. Garcinia cambogia attenuates diet induced adiposity but exacerbates hepatic collagen accumulation and inflammation. World J Gastroenterol 2013;19:4689–701.

42. Studzinska-Sroka E, Holderna Kedzia E, Galanty A, et al. In Vitro antimicrobial activity of extracts and compounds isolated from cladonia uncicalis. Nat Prod Res 2015;29:2303–7.

43. Sokolov DN, Zarubaev VV, Shtro AA, et al. Anti-viral activity of (-)- and (+)-usnic acids and their derivatives against influenza virus a (H1N1). Bioorg Med Chem 2012;22:7060–4.

44. Su ZQ, Mo ZZ, Liao JB, et al. Usnic acid protects LPS-induced acute lung injury in mice through attenuating inflammatory responses and oxidative stress. Int Immunopharmacol 2014;22:371–8.

45. Han D, Matsumaru K, Rettori D, et al. Usnic acid induced necrosis of cultures mouse hepatocytes: inhibition of mitochondrial function and oxidative stress. Biochem Pharmacol 2014;67:439–51.
46. Araujo AAS, deMelo MGD, Rabelo TK, et al. Review of the biological properties and toxicity of usnic acid. Nat Prod Res 2015;6419:1–14.
47. Lee AY, Jang Y, Hong S, et al. Ephedrine-induced mitophagy via oxidative stress in human hepatic stellate cells. J Toxicol Sci 2017;42(4):461–73.
48. Strahl S, Ehret V, Dahm HH, et al. Necrotising hepatitis after taking herbal remedies. Dtsch Med Wochenschr 1998;123:1410–4.
49. Stickel F, Baumuller HM, Seitz KH, et al. Hepatitis induced by kava kava (piper methysticum rhizome). J Hepatol 2003;39:62–7.
50. Nerurkar PV, Dragull K, Tang Cs. In vitro toxicity of kava alkaloid, pipermethystine, in HepG2 cells compared to kavalactones. Toxicol Sci 2004;79(1):106.
51. Fluyay D, Revadigar N. Biochemical benefits, diagnosis, and clinical risks evaluation of kratom. Front Psychiatry 2017;8:62.
52. Riverso M, Chang M, Soldevilla-Picco C, et al. Histologic characterization of kratom use-associated liver injury. Gastroenterol Res 2018;11(1):79–82.
53. Osborne CS, Overstreet AN, Rockey DC, et al. Drug-induced liver injury caused by kratom use as an alternative pain treatment amid an ongoing opioid epidemic. J Investig Med High Impact Case Rep 2019;7. 2324709619826167.
54. Liu J, Pei M, Zheng C, et al. A systems-pharmacology analysis of herbal medicines used in health improvement treatment: predicting potential new drugs and targets. Evid Based Complement Alternat Med 2013;2013:938764.
55. Stickel F, Droz S, Patsenker E, et al. Severe hepatotoxicity following ingestion of Herbalife contaminated with Bacillus subtilis. J Hepatol 2009;50:111–7.
56. Miller GM, Streipp R. A study of western pharmaceuticals contained within samples of Chinese herbal/patent medicines collected from New York City's Chinatown. Leg Med (Tokyo) 2007;9:258–64.
57. Gurley BJ, Gardner SF, Hubbard MA. Content versus label claims in ephedra-containing dietary supplements. Am J Health Syst Pharm 2000;57:963–9.
58. DSHEA, chapter III, Major issued and Recommendations related to labeling of dietary supplements. Available at: http://www.health.gov/dietsupp/ch3.htm. Accessed March 26, 2019.
59. Kapetanovic IM, Crowell JA, Krishnaraj R, et al. Exposure and toxicity of green tea polyphenols in fasted and non-fasted dogs. Toxicology 2009;260:28–36.
60. Cirulli ET, Nicoletti P, Abramson K, et al. A missense variant in PTPN22 is a risk factor for drug induced liver injury. Gastroenterology 2019;156(6):1707–16.e2.
61. Park SY, Viray M, Johnston D, et al. Acute hepatitis and liver failure following the use of a dietary supplement intended for weight loss or muscle building- May-October 2013. MMWR Morb Mortal Wkly Rep 2013;62(40):817–9.
62. Zheng EX, Rossi S, Fontana RJ, et al. Risk of liver injury associated with green tea extract in SLIMQUICK(®) weight loss products: results from the DILIN Prospective study. Drug Saf 2016;39(8):749–54.
63. Yang L, Aronsohn A, Hart J, et al. Herbal hepatoxicity from Chinese skullcap: a case report. World J Hepatol 2012;4:231–3.
64. Elinav E, Pinsker G, Safadi R, et al. Association between consumption of Herbalife nutritional supplements and acute hepatotoxicity. J Hepatol 2007;47:514–20.
65. Araujo JL, Worman HJ. Acute liver injury associated with a newer formulation of the herbal weight loss supplement Hydroxycut. BMJ Case Rep 2015;2015 [pii: bcr2015210303].

Moving?

Make sure your subscription moves with you!

To notify us of your new address, find your **Clinics Account Number** (located on your mailing label above your name), and contact customer service at:

Email: **journalscustomerservice-usa@elsevier.com**

800-654-2452 (subscribers in the U.S. & Canada)
314-447-8871 (subscribers outside of the U.S. & Canada)

Fax number: 314-447-8029

Elsevier Health Sciences Division
Subscription Customer Service
3251 Riverport Lane
Maryland Heights, MO 63043

*To ensure uninterrupted delivery of your subscription,
please notify us at least 4 weeks in advance of move.

Printed and bound by CPI Group (UK) Ltd, Croydon, CR0 4YY

03/10/2024

01040406-0016